HEALING WHAT HIDES
IN THE SHADOWS

A Private Journey Through Sexual Trauma Recovery

Tools, Truth, and Hope for Survivors

Agenna Mathley

JAMKHO

Published by JAMKHO

ISBN: 979-8-9931361-0-3 (paperback)

ISBN: 979-8-9931361-2-7

ISBN:979-8-9931361-3-4 (sage edition)

First Edition

Library of Congress Control Number: 2025918677

This book is not intended as a substitute for professional mental health care. Readers are encouraged to consult a qualified, trauma-informed therapist or counselor for personalized support. For crisis resources, see the Important Notice for Readers and the resource list at the back of the book, or call 988 or text HOME to 741741.

Printed in the United States of America

For permissions, contact agenna@agennamathley.com

Dedication

To my beloved family, whose love has made this possible

To JIM — YOUR unwavering support has made me feel deeply cherished every single day. You stepped in to carry responsibilities, anticipated my needs before I even realized them, and read every word of this book twice (a true labor of love for someone who doesn't enjoy reading). You took on extra roles, joined me in countless back-porch evening talks, and never stopped believing in me. This book would not exist without your steady provision, encouragement, sacrifices, and the countless ways you've gone above and beyond.

To Kyra, Hannah, and Olivia, whose encouragement, pride, and champagne toasts at every milestone fill my heart with joy. I could not ask for three more wonderful daughters. Thank you for your honesty, insights and pushing me out of my comfort zone. And thank you all for standing by me during my "Where do you think you're going? Nobody's leaving. Nobody's walking out on this fun, old-fashioned family Christmas" moments.

To my parents, I have been able to count on you my entire life and through this process was no different. Thank you for giving me a solid foundation, unwavering support and love—and Mom, thank you for being my first editor.

To Katherine, whose late-night talks, honest insight, and commitment to my success pushed me forward. You were the first to hear about this endeavor and have been a constant prayer warrior and cheerleader with complete truth and wisdom ever since.

To Elissa, who graciously stepped in to help with editing when I finally felt ready to share this work—your fresh eyes and care meant so much.

To Jody, half a century of friendship and memories. This book carries a piece of the love you have poured into my life.

To Every Survivor

To you, reading this in secret, carrying invisible wounds –

Your pain is real. Your story matters. Your healing is possible.

And to those who didn't survive –

we carry your memory, honor the healing you deserved, and hold space for all that was left unfinished.

Contents

Important Notice for Readers

This book contains frank discussions of sexual abuse, trauma responses, and healing. While I've written it to be as supportive and gentle as possible, some content may be emotionally activating.

Please remember:

You control the pace of your reading.

It's okay to skip chapters that feel too intense.

Taking breaks is self-care, not weakness.

Grounding techniques are available in Chapter 1.

Crisis resources are listed in the back of the book.

If you're in crisis:

Call 988, text HOME to 741741, or contact emergency services.

This book is not a substitute for professional mental health care. Please consider working with a trauma-informed therapist alongside reading this book.

Introduction: Your Journey to Healing

The Case for Healing — Even if you are doing this alone.

L ISTEN. BEFORE WE GO any further, I need you to hear something: healing is real, and it's possible for you. Even if you're reading this under your covers with a flashlight. Even if you've never told a soul. Even if that voice in your head keeps saying you're too damaged or it's been too long or you should've gotten over it by now.

If you're carrying sexual trauma, you already know it doesn't just go away. It's there when your shoulders tense up for no reason. It's there when relationships feel like walking through a minefield. It's there in that constant, exhausting feeling that you're somehow different from everyone else—like you're faking being okay while inside everything's falling apart.

I get it. It's like being an actor in your own life, playing the part of "normal person" while the real you is drowning.

But here's what I've learned, and what science proves: your brain and body remember how to heal. They're actually designed for it. Through small things—learning breathing exercises that actually work, moving your body in ways that feel safe, making art, journaling, learning to say no, finding just one person who gets it—you can start letting go of pain that's been stuck inside you for way too long.

Listen to me: You are not what happened to you. You are not ruined. You are not broken. You are someone who survived something that no one should have to survive, and you are brave enough to be reading these words right now. Do you know how much courage that takes?

Why Don't You Feel Like Yourself Anymore?

Something happened, and ever since, you've felt... off. Like you're wearing a costume that doesn't quite fit. Maybe you can pinpoint the exact moment everything changed. Maybe it's more like a fog that rolled in slowly until one day you realized you couldn't see yourself anymore.

That constant tension in your body? That feeling like you're watching your life from outside yourself? That sadness that sits on your chest like a weight? Those aren't flaws or weaknesses. They're your body waving a red flag saying, "Hey, we're still carrying something we shouldn't have to carry. We need help here."

Here's what pisses me off: In America, we don't talk about sexual trauma. We act like it doesn't exist. While other types of abuse have (finally) gotten some airtime, sexual trauma stays wrapped in shame and secrecy. Meanwhile, survivors like you walk around feeling completely alone, like you're the only one with this secret eating you alive.

That silence? It's literally killing people. And I'm done with it.

I wrote this book because you deserve so much better than silence and shame. You deserve to be seen, to be believed, to have tools that actually help—even if you're not ready to say the words out loud yet.

What Trauma Actually Is (And Why It's Not Your Fault)

This completely changed how I understood everything: trauma isn't the bad thing that happened to you. Trauma is what got trapped inside you when the bad thing happened.

Think of it like this: When danger hits, your body floods with survival energy—to run, fight, scream, get help. But what if you couldn't run? What if you couldn't fight back? What if you froze, or you were too small, or they threatened you, or a million other reasons why you couldn't escape?

All that survival energy had nowhere to go. So it got stuck. And stuck energy doesn't just evaporate—it transforms into depression that feels like drowning in slow motion. Into anxiety that ambushes you out of nowhere, or hurting yourself because physical pain feels easier than emotional pain. It is addictions that promise escape but deliver more chains. That energy causes mystery pain at which doctors shrug, or serious health issues like heart problems, autoimmune diseases, even cancer. It gives you that creeping feeling you're gonna die young (because yeah, trauma literally affects your lifespan).

Right now it might look like being constantly on edge, feeling cut off from everyone who loves you, or completely losing it over something "small." This isn't weakness. This is literally how trauma rewires your brain and body.

But here's the hope: starting to heal—even the tiniest baby steps—can break this cycle. You don't have to feel ready. You don't have to feel brave. You just have to be willing to try one small thing. That's it.

The Hard Truth About Who Hurts Us

This is the part that makes everything so much harder: about 93% of kids who are sexually abused are hurt by someone they know. About a third of the time, it's actually a family member—an uncle, older cousin, stepparent, someone who was supposed to keep you safe.

This is why it's all so complicated. Why you might still love someone who hurt you. Why holidays can make you want to disappear. Why trusting anyone feels like stepping off a cliff blindfolded.

But listen—that betrayal, as deep as it goes, doesn't get the final word on who you are or what you deserve. It doesn't.

Who This Book Is For

This book is for you if something sexual happened that shouldn't have—and deep down, you know it. It's for you if you're ready to try some gentle ways to feel better, even if you're scared. It's for you if you're in your 20s, 30s, or 40s or beyond and still carrying old pain. It's for you if you want real tools that work with or without therapy. And it's for you if you need to do this quietly, privately, at your own speed.

Not sure exactly what happened? That's okay too. This book won't push you to dig up memories or remember things you're not ready for. But if reading brings up unexpected stuff, please—reach out to someone safe. A counselor, a hotline, someone. Your safety comes first, always.

Why This Book Exists

You might have picked up this book for several reasons. Maybe you know something happened, but you've never told anyone. Maybe you're tired of pretending you're fine. You want to heal but can't imagine telling anyone. Or you're starting to realize that what happened is affecting you more than you thought.

Here's what I need you to know: You don't have to tell anyone to start healing. You don't have to have perfect memories. You don't have to know exactly what to call what happened to you. You just have to be willing to start.

Why This Hurts So Much — And Why Healing Is Worth It

Sexual trauma doesn't just mess with your emotions—it literally rewires your brain. Your amygdala (think of it as your brain's smoke detector) gets jammed in the "DANGER! DANGER!" position. It won't stop screaming even when you're safe. Meanwhile, your prefrontal cortex (the logical, planning, "I can handle this" part) basically goes offline when you're stressed.

That's why you feel foggy. Why you can't focus. Why you don't trust your own judgment. It's not a character flaw—it's your nervous system still stuck in protection mode from something that already happened.

All that trapped survival energy? It's still in there. It shows up as panic attacks that come from nowhere. Stomach problems that won't quit.

Unexplained pain everywhere. Feeling numb, checked out, not really here. Shame so heavy it's hard to breathe. Saying yes when you mean no until you forget what you actually want. Anger that surprises even you. Being terrified of getting close to anyone. Feeling like an alien in your own body.

This is "the body keeping the score"—trauma lives everywhere, not just in your head.

But here's the game-changer: the same body holding all this pain also holds your ability to heal. Through movement, finding your voice, breathing in new and helpful ways, creating safety—you can release what's trapped. Healing doesn't mean pretending it never happened. It doesn't mean you have to forgive anyone. It means taking back your life with tools you didn't have before.

You were never supposed to carry this forever. Can you imagine—even for a second—what it might feel like to set down even one piece of this weight?

Don't Be Angry at Your Symptoms — Listen to Them

I know. Some days you probably hate your body for how it reacts. The panic, the tension, all the ways you feel broken. But what if these symptoms aren't trying to punish you? What if they're actually trying to help?

Your symptoms are your body's way of saying: "Something hurt us. We're still holding it. We need care." They're not your enemy. They're messengers.

Here's what trauma might look like in your everyday life:

In Your Body: Constant pain or tension (hello, daily headaches and clenched jaw). Sleep? What's sleep? Nightmares that make you dread bedtime. Spacing out, feeling floaty, not quite real. Jumpiness, always waiting for the other shoe to drop. Can't stand being touched OR need touch desperately.

In Your Mind and Heart: Anxiety attacks that hijack your whole day. Intrusive thoughts and memories you can't shake. Rage that feels too big for your body. Sadness that weighs a thousand pounds. Shame whispering cruel lies about who you are. Trust issues that push everyone away. Feeling worthless, ruined, beyond repair.

Recognizing these? That's not weakness. That's the first brave step toward getting better.

What Healing Actually Means

Healing doesn't mean you'll forget what happened. It doesn't mean you'll never be triggered. It doesn't mean you have to forgive anyone. Healing means your past stops controlling your present, you can feel safe in your own body, triggers become less intense and less frequent, you develop healthy ways to manage difficult emotions, relationships become possible (even beautiful), and you reclaim parts of yourself that went into hiding.

This healing is possible without ever telling your story out loud. Your body knows what happened. Your nervous system remembers. And with the right tools, you can release what's been trapped—privately, safely, at your own pace.

How to Use This Book

This book is designed for private healing. Every tool, every exercise, and every practice can be done alone. You won't find pressure to "tell someone" or "report it" or "confront your abuser." Some survivors find these steps helpful, but your path to healing is uniquely yours.

Instead, you'll find body-based practices that release trapped trauma. You will discover ways to recognize and change trauma patterns. You will get tools for managing triggers and flashbacks, and strategies for building safety in your body. It will provide guidance for navigating relationships, and finally, hope that healing is possible.

Some chapters might feel more relevant than others. Some exercises might work better for you. That's perfect. This is your journey, at your pace, in your way.

What This Book Is (And Isn't)

Real talk: this book isn't therapy. It can't replace working with a good counselor. What it is: a toolbox full of gentle, actually-works strategies to help you start feeling better. Whether you're in therapy or not. Whether you've told someone or not. Whether you have support or you're going solo.

Think of this as your companion for the messy middle—that space between where you are now (hurting) and where you want to be (healing). If you can get therapy, absolutely do it. But if you're not there yet, these tools can still make a real difference.

A Note on Perspective and Limitations

I want to be transparent with you from the start: This book was written from my perspective as a white woman who experienced trauma in a specific context. The principles of healing I share are based on proven trauma research conducted with people across all races, cultures, and backgrounds, and years of working with survivors from diverse communities. However, I recognize that trauma healing can look different across cultures, communities, and identities, and your healing journey may include elements that aren't reflected in my particular experience.

The tools and principles in this book can help anyone heal from trauma. However, I cannot fully speak to the unique challenges that survivors from different racial, ethnic, or cultural backgrounds may face. These challenges might include navigating systems that weren't designed for them, cultural barriers to seeking help, and additional layers of healing needed from collective and historical trauma.

If you're reading this as a person of color, as someone from a marginalized community, or as someone whose experience differs from mine, these tools can still support your healing journey. I also encourage you to seek additional resources that speak to your specific cultural context and address the unique aspects of your experience that this book may not fully cover.

Your Voice in This Process

As you read, I encourage you to trust your instincts about what feels right for your situation, adapt everything to fit your cultural context and personal needs, seek culturally affirming support when you're ready for additional help, and honor your own wisdom about what your healing journey should look like.

Your experience is valid. Your cultural perspective matters. And your path to healing, whatever it looks like, deserves to be honored and supported.

A Note About Courage

If you're reading this, you've already shown incredible courage. Not the loud, visible kind that gets celebrated. But the quiet courage of surviving each day with this secret, functioning despite the weight you carry, seeking healing even when hope feels dangerous, and opening this book when part of you wanted to run.

That courage is enough. You don't need more. You just need to take one small step, then another.

You're Not Alone

One in three girls and one in six boys experience sexual abuse before age 18. Many never tell anyone. You're not alone in your silence. You're not alone in your struggle. You're not alone in your hope for something better.

The journey ahead isn't about becoming someone new. It's about uncovering who you've always been underneath the trauma. It's about teaching your body that the danger has passed. It's about reclaiming the life that's been waiting for you.

The Case for Healing — One Last Time

You don't have to stay stuck in this pain. You don't have to white-knuckle through life forever. You don't have to do this alone, even if your story stays private for now.

Healing matters because YOU matter. *You are valuable beyond measure and loved more than words can describe.* All that trapped energy—the fear, the shame, the disconnect—it can shift. Not instantly. Not perfectly. But little by little, breath by breath, one brave choice at a time.

Every small thing you try from this book counts. Every time you breathe through panic instead of letting it win. Every boundary you set. Every moment you choose kindness toward yourself instead of the usual harsh judgment. It's all building something new.

You're not alone. Just by reading this, you've already started. You're already choosing differently.

What could change if you let yourself believe—just for a moment—that you could actually heal?

Only one way to find out. Take a breath. Turn the page when you're ready. We're doing this together.

You survived the abuse. Now it's time to heal from the survival.

PART I: UNDERSTANDING WHAT HAPPENED

Foundational Knowledge for Your Healing Journey

1

Understanding Your Body

Your body holds both the wound and the wisdom. Healing happens when you're brave enough to listen to both.

I F YOU'VE EVER FELT like your body is a stranger to you—like it's this thing you're stuck with but don't really trust—I get it. After trauma, your body can feel like the enemy. Maybe it feels too tense, always on guard. Maybe it feels numb when you desperately want to feel something. Maybe you hate looking at it or being in it.

Here's what I want you to know: your body didn't betray you. It's been trying to protect you the only way it knows how. This chapter is about understanding why your body feels the way it does after trauma, and how to slowly, gently start making friends with it again—all on your own terms, without having to tell anyone your story.

Why Your Body Comes First in Healing

Before we dive into anything else, I need you to understand something crucial: you cannot heal trauma while your nervous system still believes you're in danger. This isn't a metaphor—it's biology.

When your body is stuck in survival mode, the parts of your brain responsible for healing, learning, and growth are literally offline. It's like trying to have a deep conversation while a fire alarm is blaring. Your brain can only focus on one thing: staying alive.

This is why we start with your body, not your thoughts or memories. This is why feeling safe in your skin matters more than understanding what happened to you. As we discussed in the introduction, trauma isn't stored in your thinking brain—it's stored in your nervous system, your muscles, your gut, and your reflexes. Your body has been protecting you by staying alert, tense, and ready for danger. Before we can process anything else, we need to help your nervous system learn that the immediate danger is over.

What Survival Mode Actually Looks Like

You might not realize you're stuck in survival mode because it can become so normal. You might not realize you're stuck in survival mode because it can become so normal. But if you experience constant alertness like you're always scanning for threats, your nervous system is still protecting you. The same is true if you have difficulty truly relaxing even in safe spaces. Overreacting to small things like loud noises or unexpected touch is another sign. So is feeling numb or like you're "not really there." People-pleasing to avoid any possibility of conflict shows your nervous system at work. Carrying the expectation that bad things will happen is also a protective response. Physical tension that never fully goes away rounds out these common survival mode experiences.

These responses aren't random—they're different parts of you that formed to handle overwhelming experiences, each trying to keep you safe in the only way they know how. These aren't character flaws. These aren't signs you're "too sensitive" or "overreacting." These are signs of a nervous system that learned to prioritize survival over everything else. And that nervous system did exactly what it was supposed to do—it kept you alive.

The Problem with Survival Mode

Survival mode saved your life during the trauma. But when it becomes your permanent operating system, it limits everything else. Learning becomes harder because your brain is focused on scanning for danger, not absorbing new information. Relationships become exhausting because you're constantly assessing threat levels instead of enjoying connection. Joy feels impossible because pleasure and safety can't coexist with hypervigilance. Your body feels like the enemy because it's holding all this tension and reactivity.

The goal isn't to "get over" trauma or "be stronger." The goal is to help your body learn that it's safe to come out of survival mode.

Why Body Awareness Is the Foundation

Everything else in this book—the exercises, the insights, the healing strategies—only works when your body feels safe enough to try them. You can't think your way out of trauma because trauma lives in your nervous system, muscles, and reflexes—not just in your thoughts.

This is why safety isn't a luxury in trauma healing—it's the foundation. You can't process trauma while your body is still bracing for impact. Healing requires your nervous system to shift from defense to openness. Your body needs to feel the safety that your mind knows intellectually.

When people say "just think positive" or "let it go," they don't understand that your body is still holding the experience. Your shoulders are still braced for the next hit. Your stomach is still clenched against the next violation. Your nervous system is still saying "DANGER" even when your mind knows you're safe.

What This Chapter Will Do

The exercises in this chapter aren't about "fixing" your body or forcing it to relax. They're about helping you recognize when you're in survival mode versus when you're actually present. They are for teaching your nervous system that it's safe to notice sensations without being overwhelmed. They will help by building tolerance for being in your body even when it feels uncomfortable, and creating experiences of safety and groundedness that your body can remember.

Some days these exercises will feel easy. Some days they'll feel impossible. Both responses give you information about what your nervous system needs.

Remember: Your body isn't broken. It's protective. And with patience and gentleness, it can learn to feel safe again.

When Trauma Gets Stuck in Your Body

You know how people say "it's all in your head"? Well, that's bullshit. Trauma doesn't just mess with your thoughts—it literally changes how your body works. Your muscles remember. Your nervous system remembers. Your gut remembers.

Think about it: when something scary happens, your whole body responds. Your heart races, your muscles tense up, you might feel sick to your stomach. With sexual abuse, all those physical responses get activated, but often there's no way to complete the survival response—no way to fight or run. So all that survival energy gets trapped in your body like a spring that's been compressed but never released.

This is why you might have chronic pain that doctors can't explain, or tension that never seems to go away. You might experience a feeling of being constantly on edge like something bad is about to happen. You may feel numbness or feeling disconnected from your body. Or, the opposite like stomach problems, headaches, and other physical symptoms with no clear cause.

For teens, this is extra complicated because your body is already changing so much. Add trauma on top of normal teenage body weirdness, and it's no wonder you might feel like your body is this alien thing you're forced to live in.

Why Your Body Matters in Healing

I know it might seem easier to just ignore your body—to live from the neck up and pretend the rest doesn't exist. A lot of survivors do this. We disconnect because connection hurts. We go numb because feeling is overwhelming.

But here's the thing: your body isn't just where the trauma got stuck. It's also where healing happens. Your body holds the key to feeling safe again, to experiencing joy again, to knowing what it feels like to be okay in your own skin.

This doesn't mean diving into pain or forcing yourself to feel things you're not ready for. It means slowly learning to listen to your body's signals again—starting with what feels neutral or even good.

Jordan's Story: Learning to Listen

Let me tell you about Jordan, who's 17 and has been dealing with the aftermath of trauma for two years.

When Jordan was 15, they got their first after-school job at a small local shop that smelled like vanilla candles and old wood. At first, it felt like freedom—their own money, independence, a chance to save for the car they'd been dreaming about. Their boss, a man in his forties with graying temples and an easy smile that made parents trust him immediately, seemed great initially. He remembered details about Jordan's day, asked about school projects, and even offered flexible hours during exam week.

But gradually, the atmosphere changed. He started making comments about how Jordan was "growing up," his eyes lingering on their body in a way that made their skin crawl. The compliments became uncomfortable—remarks about how their jeans fit, how they'd "filled out" over the summer. Then came the inappropriate touching during what he called "training sessions," his hands finding excuses to brush against Jordan's shoulders, their back, places that had nothing to do with learning how to stock shelves or work the register.

It escalated to pressure to stay late when no one else was around, the fluorescent lights humming overhead while he found reasons to stand too close, his cologne overwhelming in the small back office. Jordan froze every time, their voice disappearing, their body betraying them by going completely still instead of fighting back or walking away. When they finally quit the job, they mumbled something about needing to focus on school, their cheeks burning with shame they couldn't name.

After that, Jordan's relationship with their body went to hell. They started wearing only baggy clothes, layer after layer even in the heat, avoiding mirrors that might reflect back someone who looked "too grown up" or might somehow invite unwanted attention. Their shoulders were constantly hunched up by their ears, as if they could disappear into themselves. They got headaches that felt like a vice around their skull, tension so tight it made their jaw ache. During stressful times—tests, family dinners, whenever someone mentioned their old job—they'd completely space out, friends would wave their hands in front of Jordan's face, joking about how they'd "left the building."

Jordan thought this was just how life was now, that the constant vigilance and disconnection were permanent fixtures of being 17. Then one day, browsing through a book at the library, they came across a simple breathing exercise. Skeptical but desperate for any relief from the weight pressing on their chest, they tried it in a corner of the stacks where no one could see.

For the first time in months, they felt their shoulders drop a little. Just a little. It wasn't magic—the tension came right back as soon as they thought about it—but it was something. It was proof that their body could remember what relaxation felt like, even if only for seconds.

Slowly, Jordan started paying attention to their body in small ways. They'd notice when their stomach clenched (usually when certain songs played on the radio or when they passed the street where their old workplace sat, now with a "For Lease" sign in the window). They tried gentle stretches before bed, not to "fix" anything, but just to feel what it was like to move without judgment, to inhabit their limbs without fear.

The biggest shift came when Jordan realized their body wasn't the enemy—it was trying to protect them. That constant tension? Their body staying ready to defend them from any future threat. The spacing out? Their body's brilliant way of escaping when things felt too overwhelming to process. Understanding this helped Jordan feel less broken and more... human. Less like a malfunctioning machine and more like a person whose body was working exactly as designed to keep them safe.

How Trauma Lives in Your Body

Based on what survivors experience, here's how trauma might be showing up physically for you:

The Always-On-Guard Body shows up as shoulders constantly tense, jaw clenched without realizing it, jumping at sudden noises, heart racing for "no reason," and an inability to fully relax even when safe.

The Checked-Out Body feels numb or like you're floating, doesn't notice hunger, cold, or bathroom needs, feels disconnected during conversations, and sees a stranger when looking in mirrors.

The Body That Hurts experiences unexplained headaches, stomachaches, or back pain, feels like carrying invisible weight, has exhaustion that sleep doesn't fix, and develops physical symptoms that worsen with stress.

The Body You Can't Stand involves hating how you look, feeling "dirty" no matter how much you shower, avoiding touch even when it's safe, and feeling like your body betrayed you.

These aren't character flaws or signs you're weak. They're normal responses to abnormal situations.

Gentle Ways to Reconnect

You don't need to love your body right away. You don't even need to like it. You just need to start noticing it with curiosity instead of judgment. Here are some ways to begin:

The Three-Times Check-In: Three times a day, pause and notice one thing your body is feeling right now. Not to fix it, just to notice. "Tight shoulders." "Tired eyes." "Comfortable in this chair." That's it. Try setting a reminder on your phone to help you remember.

Grounding: When you feel disconnected, try one of the following grounding approaches.

5-4-3-2-1 Technique: name five things you can see, four you can hear, three you can touch, two you can smell, and one you can taste.
Categories: List as many items as you can in any three categories. Categories include movies, animals, colors, and more.

Mental exercises: Trycounting backwards, naming objects around you, spelling items you see.

Movement Without Goals: Put on music and move however feels good—or just okay. Not exercise, not dance, just movement. Let your body do whatever it wants. Stop whenever you want.

The Shower Reset: In the shower, pay attention to the water temperature on different parts of your body. Notice without judging. This reconnects you to physical sensation in a safe, private way.

Breathing Like You Mean It: Breathe in for four counts, hold for four counts, out for six counts. Put your hand on your belly and feel it move. This tells your nervous system you're safe right now.

Safe Touch Exploration: If it feels okay, try gentle self-touch like rubbing lotion on your arms, massaging your scalp, hugging yourself, or wrapping in a soft blanket. Always do this with your own consent. Stop if it feels wrong at any time.

Body Awareness: Sexual abuse often creates disconnection from your body as a protective mechanism. If you feel numb or "outside your body" while reading this chapter, the body awareness practices can help you stay grounded and present.

NEED MORE SUPPORT? EXPANDED BODY INVENTORY

For readers who feel disconnected from physical sensations

If you're reading this expanded version, you may be someone who feels "numb," "empty," or like you're "floating outside your body." This is incredibly common for sexual abuse survivors. Your nervous system learned to disconnect from your body as a protective mechanism. There's nothing wrong with you - your body was being wise.

What disconnection might feel like: "I can't feel anything below my neck," "It's like I'm watching myself from above," "My body feels like it belongs to someone else," "I only feel emotions in my head, not my body," or "I bump into things because I don't know where my body ends."

Preparing for Body Awareness

Safety Check: Before we begin, establish safety. Are you in a private space where you won't be interrupted? Do you have a trusted person you can contact if needed? Can you stop this exercise at any time without consequence? Do you have a grounding object nearby like a soft blanket or stress ball?

Permission Setting: Say to yourself (out loud if possible): "I give myself permission to feel what I feel, or to feel nothing at all. Both are okay. I am in control of this experience."

The Gentle Return: Step-by-Step Body Inventory

Stage 1: External Awareness (Start Here If You Feel Very Disconnected)

Step 1: Temperature Mapping - Notice the temperature of the air on your skin. Is your face warm or cool? Are your hands warmer or cooler than your face? Can you feel air moving from a fan or your breathing? If you can't feel temperature, that's information too. Your nervous system is protecting you. Just notice the absence of sensation without judgment.

Step 2: Pressure Points - Press your feet into the floor, squeeze your hands together, hug yourself gently, and sit back in your chair to feel it supporting you. External pressure can help you feel your body's boundaries when internal sensation is limited.

Step 3: Movement Awareness - Slowly move your head side to side, shrug your shoulders up and down, wiggle your fingers and toes, and rock gently back and forth. Movement creates sensation that's easier to detect than stillness.

Stage 2: Surface Sensations

Step 4: Clothing Contact - Notice where your clothes touch your skin, feel the texture of your sleeves against your arms, notice the weight of your clothing, and feel your shoes or the floor against your feet.

Step 5: Skin Sensation Exploration - Gently touch your arm with your opposite hand. Notice if it's soft, rough, warm, or cool. Try different types of touch like light brushing, gentle pressure, or circular motions. Touch different parts like hands, arms, or legs, but only where it feels safe. For those with touch trauma, start with hands only or use a soft object like a feather or silk scarf instead of direct touch.

Stage 3: Internal Landscape

Step 6: Breath as Gateway - Breathing is often the easiest internal sensation to detect. Place one hand on your chest, one on your belly. Don't change your breathing, just notice it. Which hand moves more? Can you feel the air moving in and out of your nose? Notice cool air in, warm air out.

Step 7: Heartbeat Discovery - Place your hand on your chest. Can you feel your heartbeat? (It's okay if you can't.) Try placing fingers on your wrist pulse point, or try jumping in place ten times, then check again. If you can't feel your heartbeat, this is common with dissociation. Your heart is still beating—your nervous system is just not consciously registering it.

Step 8: Internal Sensations Inventory - Go through each area slowly, with great patience.

Head and Face: Can you feel tension in your forehead, pressure behind your eyes, or jaw tightness? If numb, gently massage your temples and notice if this creates any sensation. If overwhelmed, just acknowledge "head area" and move on.

Neck and Shoulders: Can you feel the weight of your head, muscle tension, or warmth and coolness? If numb, roll your shoulders slowly and notice any sensation from movement. If painful, breathe into the area without trying to change it.

Arms and Hands: Can you feel energy in your arms, tingling in fingertips, or heaviness and lightness? If numb, clap your hands together and notice the sound and vibration. If disconnected, look at your hands and remind yourself "these are my hands."

Chest and Heart: Can you feel expansion with breath, tightness or openness, or heaviness? If numb, place both hands on your chest and feel the external warmth. If emotional, remember that emotions often live here—it's okay to feel sad, scared, or angry.

Stomach and Abdomen: Can you feel hunger, tension, butterflies, emptiness, or fullness? If numb, gently pat this area and notice if you can feel the external sensation. If triggering, this area often holds trauma—go very slowly or skip for now.

Pelvis and Hips: Can you feel contact with your chair, tension, heaviness, or openness? If numb, shift your weight from side to side in your chair. If traumatic, you can acknowledge this area exists without trying to feel it.

Legs and Feet: Can you feel weight of your legs, contact with floor, or circulation? If numb, stomp your feet gently and notice vibration traveling up your legs. If restless, movement in legs often indicates nervous system activation.

Working with What You Find

If You Feel Nothing: This is not failure. Numbness is your nervous system's way of protecting you. Say "Thank you, body, for keeping me safe." Try the external awareness exercises like temperature, pressure, and movement. Consider this progress—you're paying attention to your body, even if it's not responding yet.

If You Feel Too Much: You're not broken. Your nervous system is very sensitive right now. Use grounding like the 5-4-3-2-1 technique, cold water on wrists, or feet on floor. Go slower, take breaks between body areas. Remember you can stop anytime.

If Sensations Feel Strange or Scary: This is normal. Your body has been offline, so coming back online feels weird. You might feel tingling, electricity, floating, heaviness, hot, cold, or vibrating. Breathe through strange sensations. Don't resist the sensation—stay there with them and simply breathe. Remind yourself "These are just sensations. They will pass."

If Emotions Arise: Bodies hold emotions. As you reconnect, feelings may surface. Common emotions include sadness for lost connection, fear of feeling, or anger at what happened. Let emotions move through you—they have intelligence. You can feel emotions and stay safe at the same time.

Building Your Practice

Week 1-2: Foundation - Do this exercise every other day. Focus only on external awareness (Stages 1-2). Celebrate any sensation, however small. Track "Today I noticed..." in a journal.

Week 3-4: Expansion - Add internal awareness (Stage 3) when ready. Some days you'll feel more, some days less—both are fine. Notice patterns like what time of day works best or what position. Begin to notice how emotions affect body sensations.

Month 2 and Beyond - Your body awareness will fluctuate, and this is normal. Start noticing body signals throughout the day. Use body awareness for decision-making by asking "What does my body say about this?" Integrate with other healing practices.

Special Considerations

For Severe Dissociation: Start with just two to three minutes. Focus on external sensations only. Have someone nearby if possible. Consider working with a trauma-informed therapist.

For Specific Trauma Locations: You can skip any area that feels unsafe. Return to these areas only when you feel ready. Sometimes healing other areas first makes difficult areas accessible later. Professional support can be helpful for trauma-specific areas.

For Hypervigilance: You might feel "too much" in some areas. Practice saying "I notice this sensation, and I am safe." Alternate between areas that feel intense and areas that feel calm. Breathing helps regulate overwhelming sensations.

Affirmations for Body Reconnection

Use these as you practice: "My body is wise and has kept me alive," "I am learning to be at home in my body again," "Feeling nothing is still feeling something," "My body and I are becoming friends again," "I trust my body's timing for healing," and "Each moment of awareness is a victory."

When to Seek Additional Support

Consider professional help if: You consistently feel unsafe during this exercise. Flashbacks or panic attacks occur regularly. You feel completely unable to sense your body after several weeks. Practicing body awareness triggers urges to self-harm, or you need guidance working with trauma-specific areas.

Remember: Reconnecting with your body after trauma is one of the bravest things you can do. Your body has been waiting patiently for you to come home. Take your time, be gentle, and trust the process.

Working with Resistance

Sometimes when you try to connect with your body, it feels scary or overwhelming. That's okay. Your body learned to protect itself by disconnecting, and it might not trust you yet.

If exercises feel too much, make them smaller like checking in once a day instead of three times. Try for just ten seconds, focus on neutral body parts like your elbows or ears, and remember you can stop anytime. The goal isn't to push through resistance—it's to gently work with it.

Why This Matters

Your body has been carrying you through one of the hardest things a person can experience. It's been protecting you the best way it knows how, even when that protection feels uncomfortable or painful.

Learning to understand and work with your body—instead of against it—is a huge part of healing. Not because you need to "fix" anything, but because you deserve to feel at home in your own skin again.

As established earlier, one in three girls and one in six boys experience sexual abuse. Many of them feel disconnected from their bodies just like you might. You're not alone in this struggle, and you're not alone in the journey back to yourself.

A Final Thought

Your body is not your enemy. It's your fiercest protector, your constant companion, and eventually, it can be your friend again. Every time you notice a sensation without judgment, every time you breathe deeply, every time you choose gentle movement over numbness—you're telling your body: "I'm listening. We're safe now. We're in this together." You don't have to rush this. You don't have to be perfect at it. You just have to start, one tiny moment of awareness at a time.

Your body has kept you alive through trauma. Now it's ready to help you truly live again. Trust the process, trust your pace, and most of all, trust yourself. You've got this.

Coaching Corner: Your Body Is Wiser Than You Think

*I want you to try something right now. Put your hand on your heart and take one breath. Just one. Did you feel that? That heartbeat under your palm? That's been there through everything - every moment of trauma, every sleepless night, every day you didn't think you could keep going. Your heart just kept beating. Your body just kept working to keep you alive. I see so many survivors come into my office apologizing for their body's responses. "I should have fought back." "I shouldn't feel this way." "My body is broken." **But sitting here with you, I don't see broken. I see brilliant.** Your body made split-second decisions that kept you breathing, kept your heart pumping, kept you here so we could have this conversation today. You don't have to love your body tomorrow. But maybe, just maybe, you can stop being quite so angry at it. It's been on your team this whole time.*

2

What Is Sexual Abuse and Why It's Not Your Fault

The only person responsible for abuse is the abuser. Always.

Staying Grounded While Reading

Sexual abuse often creates disconnection from your body as a protective mechanism. If you feel numb or "outside your body" while reading this chapter, the body awareness practices from Chapter 1 can help you stay grounded and present.

Q UICK GROUNDING REMINDER: FEEL your feet on the floor, take three deep breaths, and know you can take breaks anytime you need them.

If you're reading this with a knot in your stomach, wondering if what happened to you "counts" as abuse, or if you're carrying guilt about something that was done TO you—take a breath. This chapter is about understanding what sexual abuse really is and releasing the blame you never should have carried.

The most important reframe is this: instead of asking what's wrong with survivors, we ask what happened to them. Children get hurt twice—once by the abuse and again by being left alone to make sense from senselessness.

What Sexual Abuse Actually Is

Sexual abuse is when someone uses power, control, or manipulation to violate your sexual boundaries. It's any sexual act or behavior that you didn't want, couldn't consent to, or that made you feel unsafe. This includes unwanted touching of private areas, being forced or coerced into sexual acts, someone exposing themselves to you, being shown pornographic material, sexual comments that made you uncomfortable, someone taking sexual photos of you, being manipulated into sexual behavior through "games" or "secrets," any sexual contact between an adult and child, and sexual activity between children with a power imbalance.

The key word here is POWER. Abuse is always about someone using their power—physical, emotional, age-related, or positional—to take what they want regardless of your wellbeing.

It might have happened once or hundreds of times. It might have been violent or seemingly "gentle." It might have been a stranger, but more often it's someone known and trusted. None of these details change this truth: it was abuse, and it was not your fault.

Why You Feel Like It's Your Fault (But It's Not)

If there's one thing abusers do expertly, it's convince victims they're to blame. This isn't accidental—it's how abusers protect themselves. But let's look at why your brain might have accepted responsibility for something that was never yours to carry.

The Control Illusion

Your brain desperately wants to believe you had control because that feels safer than accepting you were powerless. "If I caused it, I can prevent it." But this is a protective illusion. You didn't cause it. You couldn't have prevented it.

The Grooming Effect

Abusers are master manipulators. They plant lies like seeds that grow into self-blame: "You wanted this," "This is our special secret," "This is how people show love," "You're so mature for your age," "No one will believe you," and "This is your fault for wearing that, being here, or leading me on."

These lies burrow deep, especially in young minds trying to make sense of confusion and violation.

The Survival Brain

During abuse, your survival brain takes over. If you froze instead of fighting, didn't scream, "went along with it," felt physical sensations, returned to the abuser, or kept the secret—these were all survival strategies, not consent. Your brain did what it needed to do to keep you as safe as possible in an unsafe situation.

Understanding the Freeze Response

Since this comes up again in a later chapter, let me touch on it briefly here: the freeze response is as natural as fight or flight. When your brain calculates that fighting or running would make things worse, it shuts down your ability to move or speak. This is pure biology, not weakness.

If you froze, your brain made a split-second survival decision. This freeze response protected you from potentially worse harm, is experienced by up to 70% of assault survivors, has nothing to do with consent, and is evidence of a functioning survival system, not a character flaw.

The Truth About Responsibility

Let's be crystal clear about where responsibility actually lies. The abuser is 100% responsible because they chose to violate boundaries, knew it was wrong (hence the secrecy), used their power to take what they wanted, and created the entire situation.

You are 0% responsible, even if you didn't fight or scream, your body responded, you kept it secret, you "should have known better," you went back, or you initiated contact later.

Children and adolescents cannot consent to sexual activity with adults or with someone who has power over them. Period. Your survival responses were not participation. Your silence was not agreement. Your body's reactions were not permission.

Why This Feels Like Your Fault: The "Name It to Tame It" Principle

Shame thrives in silence and vagueness. When we can't name what we're experiencing, it feels bigger and more powerful. But when we name it—"This is shame talking" or "That's a trauma response"—we begin to tame its power over us.

Common shame-based thoughts after abuse include feeling dirty, damaged, or broken; worrying that no one will want you if they know; believing you should have stopped it; wondering if maybe you wanted it; and thinking you're making too big a deal of this.

Name these for what they are: lies that trauma tells. They're not truth. They're not you. They're the voice of unprocessed hurt.

The Many Faces of Self-Blame

Survivors blame themselves in countless creative ways, but each form of self-blame has a truth that counters it.

"I should have known better" - Knowledge doesn't equal power when you're being overpowered. You did the best you could with what you knew and the options you had.

"I didn't say no clearly enough" - The absence of a clear "no" is not a "yes," especially when fear, power dynamics, or freeze responses are involved.

"My body responded" - Physical arousal during abuse is a biological response, like crying when cutting onions. It's not consent, enjoyment, or participation.

"I went back/didn't avoid them" - Trauma bonds, grooming, and survival needs are powerful. Returning to an abuser doesn't mean you wanted abuse.

"Others have had it worse" - Pain isn't a competition. Your experience matters regardless of what others have endured.

Breaking Free from False Responsibility

Moving from self-blame to truth is a journey, not a moment. Here are some ways to begin.

Challenge the Lies: When shame thoughts arise, ask yourself, "Would I blame a friend who told me this happened to them?" "What would I say to a child experiencing this?" "Whose voice is this—mine or my abuser's?"

Practice Truth Statements: Even if you don't believe them yet, try saying, "What happened to me was abuse." "I did what I needed to do to survive." "The shame belongs to the person who hurt me," and "My survival responses were not consent."

Body-Based Relief: Shame lives in the body, so try gentle movement to discharge stuck energy, breathing exercises to calm your nervous system, and the somatic exercises you'll learn in Chapter 6.

Write It Out: Put your self-blame on paper, then write the truth next to each statement. Seeing the contrast helps your brain recognize the lies. Chapter 12 will give you specific writing exercises for healing.

What You Can Do Right Now

You might not be ready to challenge every self-blaming thought today, and that's okay. Healing happens in layers. For now, notice when you blame yourself—just noticing is powerful. Try one truth statement like "This was not my fault." Practice the "Name It to Tame It" principle by recognizing "That's shame talking, not truth." And be patient with yourself—these beliefs took time to form, so they'll take time to shift.

A Truth to Hold Onto

Sexual abuse is theft. The abuser stole your safety, your innocence, your right to develop naturally. But they could not steal your worth, your future, or your capacity to heal.

The responsibility for what happened lies entirely with the person who chose to hurt you. Not with child-you, who couldn't protect your-self. Not with frozen-you, whose body was trying to survive. Not with silent-you, who carried secrets too heavy to speak.

You deserved protection and didn't get it. *You deserved safety* and it was stolen. But *you still deserve healing*, and that's something no one can take from you.

Coaching Corner: Releasing What Was Never Yours

Close your eyes for a moment and imagine yourself at the age when the abuse happened. What would you say to that younger you? Would you blame them? Would you list all the things they "should" have done differently?

Of course not. You'd probably want to wrap them in the biggest hug and tell them none of this was their fault.

That compassion you'd show to younger you? That's the truth. Everything else—all the shame, blame, and "shoulds"—those are lies that attached themselves to your truth.

You've been carrying responsibility that was never yours to hold. It's okay to set it down. It's okay to be angry at the person who hurt you instead of at yourself. It's okay to finally put the shame where it belongs—with them, not you.

Take a breath. Feel your feet on the ground. You're here, you survived, and you're finally learning the truth: it was never, ever your fault.

3

What is Trauma?

"Trauma isn't what happened to you. It's what happened inside you because of what happened to you." Dr. Gabor Maté

I F YOU KNOW THAT someone touched you, used you, or violated you sexually when you were young—but you've been telling yourself "it wasn't that bad" or "I'm fine" or "that was so long ago"—this chapter is for you. You know what happened. What you might not know is that you're carrying trauma.

Here's the truth that changes everything: trauma isn't the bad thing that happened. Trauma is what your body and brain did to help you survive it—and what they are still doing now, years later, even though the danger has passed.

It's Not What Happened, It's What Is Still Happening

When people hear "trauma," they often think it means the event itself—the abuse, the violation, the betrayal. But trauma is actually the energy that got trapped in your nervous system when you couldn't fight or flee. It's the adaptations your brain made to keep you safe. It's the way your body learned to brace for danger. It's why you jump at loud noises, why certain smells make you sick, why you can't trust people, why you feel numb or overwhelmed for "no reason."

The event is over. But your body hasn't gotten the message yet.

Why "Just Get Over It" Doesn't Work

Think about it this way: if someone breaks your arm and it heals wrong, you don't just have a memory of a broken arm. You have an arm that doesn't work right. It hurts when it rains. It can't lift what it used to. The break happened years ago, but the impact is now.

Sexual abuse in childhood or adolescence is like that, except it affects your entire nervous system. When someone violated your boundaries—especially when you were young and dependent—your body had to adapt to survive. Those adaptations include hypervigilance (always watching for danger), dissociation (checking out when things get intense), emotional numbing or overwhelming emotions, physical tension or chronic pain, difficulty with trust and relationships, and shame that feels like it's welded to your identity.

These aren't personality defects—they're survival strategies. They're proof that your body did whatever it took to keep you alive. But now these survival strategies might be making life harder than it needs to be.

The Two-Part Definition of Trauma

Part 1: The Violation Yes, what happened to you matters. Whether it was inappropriate touching that made you uncomfortable, being forced to do things you didn't understand, someone using your body for their gratification, being exposed to sexual content too young, or any unwanted sexual experience—these violations matter because they crossed boundaries that should have been sacred. They introduced you to experiences your developing brain wasn't ready to process.

Part 2: The Ongoing Impact But trauma lives in the second part—in how your nervous system reorganized itself around the violation. It's the way your body learned to freeze instead of fight, how your brain decided trusting people was dangerous, the shame that attached itself to your identity, the ways you learned to disconnect from your body, and the protective strategies that now keep you isolated.

This is why two people can experience similar events but have different levels of trauma. It's not about comparing whose abuse was "worse." It's about how each nervous system adapted to survive.

Your Body Kept Score (Even If Your Mind Forgot)

Many survivors say things like "I can barely remember it, so why does it still affect me?", "My mind knows it wasn't my fault, but I still feel ashamed," and "I've forgiven them, so why am I still struggling?"

This confusion happens because trauma isn't stored in the thinking part of your brain. It's stored in your body, in your nervous system, in the part of your brain that controls survival. You can't think your way out of trauma any more than you can think your way out of a broken bone.

Your body remembers through physical reactions to triggers, emotional responses that seem "too big," relationship patterns that keep repeating, health issues with no clear cause, and a nervous system stuck in alarm mode.

The Hidden Nature of Sexual Trauma

Sexual trauma carries unique challenges that make it particularly complex to heal from.

Shame and Silence: Unlike other traumas, sexual abuse often comes wrapped in shame so thick you might have never spoken about it. This silence allows trauma to grow roots.

Betrayal: Often the person who hurt you was someone who should have protected you. This double wound—abuse plus betrayal—creates complex trauma.

Developmental Impact: When abuse happens during childhood or adolescence, it disrupts normal development. You might have learned that your body isn't yours, love and pain go together, you're only valuable for what others can take from you, and safety is an illusion.

Body Betrayal: Sometimes bodies respond physically during abuse. This biological response creates profound confusion and shame, even though it has nothing to do with consent or desire.

How Trauma Reorganizes the Self

When trauma happens, especially during childhood, our minds don't just store the experience as a single memory. Instead, something remarkable happens: our psyche creates internal compartments to help us survive.

Your mind creates separate compartments to hold overwhelming experiences—like having different drawers for different types of memories and feelings. The scared feelings go in one drawer, the "everything's fine" feelings in another, the anger in yet another. This allows you to function day-to-day while keeping the most overwhelming parts safely contained.

This creates what trauma specialists call "parts"—different aspects of yourself that formed to handle different pieces of an impossible situation. You might have a part that tries to stay strong, a part that still feels like the scared child, a part that learned to please everyone to stay safe, or a part that shuts down when things get overwhelming.

This isn't a sign of mental illness or weakness. It's evidence of your mind's incredible ability to survive impossible circumstances. The goal isn't to eliminate these parts but to understand them and help them work together rather than against each other.

As we explore trauma throughout this book, you'll learn to recognize these different parts of yourself, understand their protective roles, and develop relationships with them. This parts work will be essential to your healing journey, helping you integrate all aspects of yourself with compassion and understanding.

Coaching Corner: Your Body's Brilliant Protection

I want you to know something: every symptom you have, every struggle you face, every way you've adapted—they all make sense. Your body and brain did exactly what they needed to do to protect you.

That anxiety? It's your alarm system trying to keep you safe. That numbness? It protected you from overwhelming pain. That inability to trust? It made sense when trust was dangerous.

You're not broken. You're protected. And now we're going to gently update your protection system to match your current reality—where you're safe, where you have choices, and where healing is possible.

Take a breath with me. You've already survived the worst part. Now we're just teaching your body to believe it.

4

The Freeze Response in Sexual Abuse

Your body's freeze response wasn't giving up—it was giving you the best chance to survive.

I F YOU'VE SPENT YEARS haunted by the question "Why didn't I fight back?"—this chapter holds answers that might finally bring you peace. What you're about to learn could be the key to releasing the self-blame you've been carrying.

Your body did exactly what millions of years of evolution designed it to do: it kept you alive in an impossible situation. That freeze response you've been ashamed of? It's actually evidence of a perfectly functioning survival system.

Beyond Fight or Flight: The Hidden Third Response

We've all heard of "fight or flight"—the idea that when faced with danger, we either confront it or run from it. But there's a crucial third response that rarely gets talked about, especially in conversations about sexual abuse: the freeze response.

This isn't a weakness or a failure. It's an ancient survival mechanism shared by all mammals. When your brain calculates that fighting would make things worse and fleeing isn't possible, it initiates a shut-down sequence designed to maximize survival.

The Possum's Wisdom: A Story of Survival

Let me share a powerful example that shows exactly how this works in nature.

One summer night, the air thick with the sound of cicadas, my two boxer dogs were pacing near the back door, their usual evening calm replaced by excited alertness. Their ears were pricked forward, hairs bristling, and they kept pawing at the door to get out, glancing between me and the darkened yard. Something had caught their attention in the inky blackness.

Curious and slightly concerned, I let them out—and instantly, they rushed into the yard with purpose. I could hear their paws on the grass, followed quickly by frenzied barking from one dog while the other approached more cautiously, curious but clearly frightened. One dog positioned herself on one side of something on the ground, barking steadily, while the other circled at a distance, unsure but alert.

I flipped on the porch light and stepped outside, squinting as my eyes adjusted. There, illuminated in the yellow glow, was a possum. Lying completely still. Absolutely motionless. Its gray fur looked dull in the artificial light, its small black eyes stared unseeing at nothing. Clearly, it was dead. I had just been outside minutes earlier watering the garden in the fading daylight—no sign of life or death anywhere in the yard. But now this lifeless animal had somehow appeared and become the center of absolute chaos, my dogs' primitive instincts fully activated.

I called off the dogs and guided them back toward the house. My husband came out, assessed the scene and confirmed what seemed obvious: "Yeah, it's definitely dead." The possum hadn't moved a muscle despite all the noise and commotion. He went to grab work gloves and a shovel from the garage but when we returned just moments later the possum was gone. Vanished completely, as if it had never been there at all.

It hadn't been dead. It had been in immobility—a full-body freeze response so convincing that even up close, even with two agitated dogs circling and barking, we were absolutely certain it wasn't alive. That possum wasn't "playing dead"—that phrase trivializes what was actually happening. It was surviving, using an ancient biological response that shut down its entire system to avoid further danger.

Here's what matters: this isn't just a "possum thing." It's a mammalian thing. We have it too.

The Science of Tonic Immobility

When you experience overwhelming threat—especially when escape seems impossible—your nervous system can trigger the same response. Scientists call it "tonic immobility," and it involves muscle paralysis where your body literally cannot move, vocal paralysis where your voice disappears making screaming impossible, altered consciousness where you may feel disconnected or "float away," suppressed pain where your body releases chemicals to minimize suffering, and memory disruption where the experience may be stored in fragments.

Research shows that up to 70% of sexual assault survivors experience significant tonic immobility. Yet only about 5% report what happened. Why? Because our society doesn't understand the freeze response. People ask "Why didn't you fight?" without realizing that fighting wasn't an option your nervous system gave you.

The STOP Technique

S - STOP what you're doing The moment you notice you're freezing—whether your mind goes blank, you can't find words, or you feel that familiar shutdown sensation—literally stop. Don't try to push through it or force yourself to keep going. Freeze is your nervous system's way of saying "pause," so honor that signal.

T - TAKE three deep breaths Breathe slowly and deliberately. Make your exhales longer than your inhales—this activates your parasympathetic nervous system and signals safety to your body. Don't worry about breathing "perfectly." Just breathe with intention.

O - OBSERVE what's happening in your body Get curious about your internal experience without judgment. You might notice "My throat feels tight," "My chest is heavy," "I feel disconnected from my body," or "Everything feels foggy." This isn't about fixing anything yet—just noticing with compassion.

P - PAUSE before responding Give yourself permission to take time. You might say, "I need a moment to collect my thoughts," or "Let me pause here for a second." Remember: taking time to regulate isn't weakness—it's wisdom.

Breaking Free from Freeze

Remember our possum friend who shook off the freeze energy and trotted away? That possum was doing exactly what it was designed to do—complete the natural cycle and return to life. We humans have this same beautiful design wired into our nervous systems. We were created with the innate wisdom to move through stress and return to regulation, just like every other creature.

But somewhere along the way—through trauma, conditioning, or simply living in a world that doesn't honor our natural rhythms—this innate ability gets buried under layers of 'shoulds' and survival strategies. We learn to override our body's signals, to push through instead of pause, to think our way out instead of feel our way through.

The good news? This capacity for natural regulation is still there, waiting to be remembered and reclaimed. It's not broken—it's just covered up.

When you're trapped in freeze, your thinking brain goes offline. You might find yourself unable to speak, think clearly, or remember what you wanted to say. Your body is doing exactly what it's supposed to do—protecting you by shutting down until the threat passes.

But here's what the possum knew that we can remember: you have the power to signal to your nervous system that you're safe now.

The **STOP** technique gives you a way to interrupt the freeze response and begin the journey back to your regulated, thinking self. Think of it as a gentle wake-up call to your nervous system—a way to say, "Hey, I see you're trying to protect me, but I'm safe now. We can start coming back online."

The STOP technique doesn't magically solve everything, but it creates a small space between your trigger and your response. In that space, you can choose what happens next. You can choose to use one of the discharge techniques we'll explore, or simply give yourself permission to step away until you feel more grounded.

Sarah discovered this technique after years of freezing during difficult conversations with her teenage daughter. "I used to just stand there, mouth open, unable to say anything while she stormed off. Now when I feel that freeze coming on, I use STOP. I tell her, 'Honey, I love you and this conversation matters to me. Let me take a breath so I can be present with you.' It changed everything."

Why Freezing Happens During Sexual Abuse

Sexual abuse creates the perfect storm for a freeze response.

Power Imbalance: When facing someone bigger, stronger, or with authority over you, your brain instantly calculates the odds. Fighting might provoke worse violence. Running might be impossible. Freezing becomes the safest option.

Betrayal and Confusion: When abuse comes from someone you know or trust, your brain faces an impossible equation. This person is supposed to be safe, but they're hurting you. The cognitive dissonance can trigger shutdown.

Developmental Factors: Young people are especially prone to freezing because their brains are still developing threat assessment, they're socialized to comply with adults, they have limited life experience to draw from, and they're physically smaller and less powerful.

Previous Trauma: If you've experienced powerlessness before, your nervous system may default to freeze as a learned response.

Understanding the Part That Froze

When you froze during abuse, it wasn't "you" failing to fight back—it was a protective part of you making a split-second decision to keep you as safe as possible. This part, often very young, assessed the situation in milliseconds and chose the response most likely to minimize harm.

Think of this part as your body's emergency response team. When fighting seemed dangerous and fleeing seemed impossible, this part chose stillness. It's like a wise protector who knew that sometimes, being very still is the safest choice.

Many survivors carry anger at "the part that froze." But what if you could see this part differently? What if you could thank it for choosing the option that kept you alive?

Meeting Your Frozen Part Exercise: Close your eyes and imagine the part of you that froze. How old does this part seem? What does it need you to know about that moment? Can you thank this part for protecting you the best way it knew how? Tell this part: "You kept us alive. You did the right thing. We're safe now."

What Freezing Feels Like: Maria's Story

Maria was eleven when her uncle started making "special visits" to her room during family gatherings. The house would be full of cousins playing, adults laughing in the kitchen, the warm smell of her grandmother's tamales filling the air—normal family chaos that felt like a world away from what was happening behind her closed bedroom door.

She'd lie in her narrow twin bed with its faded princess sheets, hearing his heavy footsteps in the creaky hallway, the sound growing closer, and her whole body would go rigid. The familiar sounds of home—her baby cousin's laughter, the television downstairs, her mother's voice calling for someone to help set the table—would fade to a distant hum.

When he entered her room, closing the door with that soft click that meant everything was about to change, she wanted to scream for her mother, to run to the safety of the crowded living room, to push him away with all her might. But nothing worked. Her voice vanished completely, as if someone had reached down her throat and stolen it. Her limbs felt like they'd been filled with concrete, heavy and useless. She could only stare at the ceiling, at the glow-in-the-dark stars she'd stuck there during happier times, her mind floating somewhere near that plastic constellation while her body endured what felt un-endurable.

For years, Maria tortured herself with the same relentless questions: "Why didn't I fight? Why didn't I yell for help when everyone was right downstairs? Why didn't I tell my mom?" She felt like a coward, like she'd somehow "let it happen," like if she'd been braver or stronger, she could have stopped it.

But here's what was really happening: Maria's nervous system was making split-second calculations with the precision of a computer. Her uncle was bigger, stronger, and had authority in the family structure. Her parents trusted him completely—he was the favorite uncle who brought presents and made everyone laugh. Fighting might make him hurt her worse, or hurt someone else in the family. Screaming might bring everyone running, but who would believe her over the beloved uncle? Her ancient survival brain chose the option most likely to ensure survival: freeze and endure.

Maria's freeze response saved her life. It minimized physical harm. It helped her survive repeated trauma without the family unit exploding. Far from weakness, it was her nervous system's brilliant protective strategy, calibrated perfectly for an impossible situation.

The Trapped Energy Problem

Here's where humans differ from that possum: after the dogs were called off and danger passed, the possum got up, gave itself a good shake—literally discharging the freeze energy through movement—and trotted away into the night. It completed the survival cycle and moved on.

But humans often don't complete this cycle. The survival energy that helped you freeze gets stuck in your nervous system like a spring that's been compressed but never released. You survived the trauma, but your body hasn't gotten the message that it's over. This trapped energy becomes chronic anxiety or hypervigilance, depression or emotional numbness, physical pain with no clear cause, difficulty with intimacy or trust, panic attacks or flashbacks, and feeling constantly "on edge."

These aren't character flaws or signs you're broken. They're evidence that your body is still holding the charge from a threat that has passed.

Common Freeze Responses During Abuse

Understanding the various ways freeze shows up can help you recognize and validate your experience. When you are in these states, these are something you might feel.

Complete Paralysis: If you cannot move any part of your body, feel like you're made of stone, or watch what's happening like it's not real.

Partial Freeze: Some movement is possible but you feel sluggish, you can't speak but can move slightly, you feel like you're moving through molasses.

Collapsed Immobility: Your body goes completely limp, you might feel like a rag doll, and have no muscle tension at all.

Dissociative Freeze: You feel like you leave your body, watch from outside yourself, or go somewhere else in your mind.

Compliant Freeze: You go through motions without resistance, you might smile or act normal while feeling frozen inside, your body complies while mind escapes.

All of these are valid freeze responses. All of them are protection, not participation.

Releasing the Freeze: Beginning to Thaw

While the freeze response is automatic during trauma, you can help your body complete the interrupted cycle and release trapped energy.

The "Voo" Sound (Basic Version): This exercise helps discharge frozen energy from your core. Sit comfortably and take a natural breath. On the exhale, make a low "voo" sound from your belly. Let the sound vibrate through your body. Notice any warmth or tingling. Repeat 2-3 times, then rest. (You'll learn an expanded version in Chapter 6 that includes pelvic release)

Gentle Shaking: Like animals in nature who shake after escaping threat. Stand with feet hip-width apart. Begin gently bouncing your knees. Let the shaking travel up your body. Continue for 30-60 seconds. Rest and notice sensations.

Slow Movement: Frozen energy needs to move, but slowly. Make any movement extremely slowly. Notice every micro-sensation. If you feel stuck, make the movement smaller. Focus on what wants to move.

Boundary Movements: Reclaim your ability to protect yourself. Practice pushing motions with your arms. Say "no" while pushing (even whispered). Start small and build confidence. Remember: this is practice, not pressure.

Why Understanding Freeze Matters

Recognizing freeze as a legitimate survival response changes everything.

It Validates Your Experience: You weren't weak. You weren't complicit. You were surviving using an ancient, effective strategy.

It Explains Your Symptoms: Those "random" anxiety attacks? It's your body is still fighting a battle that ended years ago. Understanding this helps you approach symptoms with compassion, not judgment.

It Points to Healing: If freeze is just trapped survival energy, then healing means helping that energy complete its cycle. Your body knows how to do this—it just needs safety and support.

It Releases Shame: You can finally stop blaming yourself for not fighting back. Your nervous system made the best choice available. Period.

Moving Forward with Compassion

As you continue through this book, you'll find more tools for working with freeze responses and trapped energy. For now, practice noticing without judgment: When do you freeze in current life? What sensations accompany freezing? Can you thank your body for protecting you? What would gentle movement feel like?

Remember: your freeze response was brilliant, not broken. It kept you alive. Now, as you build safety and learn new tools, you can help your body understand that the danger has passed. The possum eventually got up and walked away. So can you.

Coaching Corner: "Your Body's Ancient Wisdom"

I want you to try something: Place your hand on your heart and say, "Thank you for protecting me."

Your body—the one you might have been angry at for "not fighting back"—did something extraordinary. In a split second, it accessed the protective instincts placed within you and chose the response most likely to keep you alive. That freeze wasn't failure. It was your body loving you the only way it knew how in that moment.

Now you're learning new ways to feel safe. But please don't dishonor the protection that saved you by calling it weakness. You survived because your body is magnificent, not because it failed you.

The same wisdom that knew to freeze then can learn to thaw now. Trust it. Trust yourself. You've been brilliant all along.

PART II: PROCESSING THE IMPACT

Working Through the Emotional Aftermath

5

Understanding and Releasing Shame

"Shame dies when stories are told in safe places." Ann Voskamp

I F YOU'RE READING THIS while a voice in your head whispers "You're disgusting," "No one would love you if they knew," or "It was your fault"—I need you to know something: that's not your voice. That's shame talking, and shame lies.

Of all the wounds sexual abuse leaves behind, shame might be the cruelest. It's the wound that convinces you that YOU are the problem, that something is fundamentally wrong with who you are. But here's the truth shame doesn't want you to know: shame belongs to the person who hurt you, not to you. This chapter is about understanding how shame attached itself to your identity and learning how to send it back where it belongs.

What Shame Really Is

Let's get clear about what we're dealing with. Shame is different from guilt. Guilt says "I did something bad" while shame says "I AM bad." Guilt can actually be helpful—it tells us when we've acted against our values. Values are your personal standards for how you want to behave. But shame attacks your very being. It doesn't just criticize what you did; it condemns who you are.

After sexual abuse, shame wraps around you like a second skin, whispering lies: "You're dirty now," "You're damaged goods," "No one will want you if they know," "You must have wanted it," and "You're different from 'normal' people."

These aren't thoughts you chose. They're psychological wounds that need healing, not character flaws that need fixing.

Shame doesn't just live in your head, either. It shows up in your body—that sick feeling in your stomach, the heat creeping up your neck, the way you want to disappear when someone looks at you. For young people especially, it hits hard because you're already trying to figure out who you are, and abuse can make you feel like you're somehow less than everyone else.

Why Sexual Abuse Creates Such Deep Shame

Sexual abuse is uniquely shame-producing for several reasons.

It Attacks Your Core: Sexuality is connected to our deepest sense of self. When someone violates these boundaries, shame attaches to your very identity.

It Happens in Secrecy: Abusers depend on secrecy, often saying things like "This is our special secret" or "No one would understand." Abusers count on shame and use it as a weapon to keep you quiet, or they make you feel like you wanted what happened. It's all designed to make you doubt yourself and stay silent.

It Confuses Responsibility: Especially when you're young, it's almost impossible to understand that someone else's actions aren't your fault. It's a normal stage of brain development where children logically conclude that if something bad happened, they must have caused it somehow. They haven't yet learned to see situations from other people's perspectives.

It May Involve Physical Responses: If your body responded during abuse, shame multiplies. But physical arousal is just biology, like your knee jerking when the doctor taps it. It has nothing to do with consent or desire.

Society Reinforces It: We live in a culture that often blames victims, asks what they were wearing, or suggests they should have fought harder. These messages deepen shame that shouldn't exist in the first place.

But here's the truth: you didn't choose any of this. The abuser did. The shame belongs to them, not you.

Why Shame Feels So Huge

Shame feels impossible to handle because it messes with how you see yourself and how you think other people see you. After abuse, you might be terrified that if anyone found out, they'd judge you or think you're disgusting. Maybe you were threatened. Maybe everyone loves the person who hurt you, and you're scared they'd take their side.

These fears make shame feel like a wall between you and the rest of the world.

Sometimes shame acts like armor—it tries to protect you by keeping your pain hidden when the world doesn't feel safe. But that same armor blocks out good things too, like friendship and love and just feeling okay in your own skin.

How Shame Shows Up in Your Life

Shame doesn't just live in your thoughts—it shapes your entire life.

In Your Body: You might find yourself avoiding mirrors, feeling "dirty" no matter how much you wash, disconnecting from physical sensations, experiencing chronic tension or feeling "heavy," wanting to hide or disappear, getting that sick feeling in your stomach, heat creeping up your neck, or feeling like your body is wrong.

In Your Relationships: Shame shows up as believing you have to earn love, accepting poor treatment because you think it's all you deserve, pushing people away before they can "find out" about you, difficulty with intimacy or trust, feeling like you're "fooling" people who think you're good, pulling away from friends, avoiding activities you used to love, or feeling like you have to be perfect all the time just to be worth anything.

In Your Daily Life: You might notice perfectionism (trying to be good enough to matter), self-sabotage when things go well, difficulty accepting compliments, feeling like an imposter, constant apologizing for existing, feeling jumpy around certain people or places, avoiding eye contact or trying to make yourself smaller.

In Your Self-Talk: Shame creates brutal inner criticism, comparing yourself to others and always falling short, minimizing your accomplishments, magnifying your mistakes, speaking to yourself in ways you'd never speak to a friend, and thinking things like "I should've said no" or "It's my fault for being there."

Those are signs that shame is trying to take over your life. But you can fight back. You didn't cause any of this—someone else made the choice to hurt you.

Real Stories of Shame

Aaliyah's Story

Let me tell you about Aaliyah, who's 14 now but was 10 when this all started.

Aaliyah's mom started dating Chris, and he seemed great at first. Funny, charming, the kind of guy who remembered to ask about school projects and always offered to help with homework. The whole family liked him—even Aaliyah's usually suspicious grandmother called him "a keeper." But when Aaliyah's mom wasn't around, the air in the room would shift, becoming thick and uncomfortable.

Chris would call Aaliyah over to sit close to him on the couch, the leather creaking under their combined weight. His hand, which seemed so normal when shaking hands with adults, would find its way to places that made Aaliyah's skin crawl. He'd touch them in ways that felt wrong and scary, his fingers leaving invisible marks that burned long after. He called it their "special game" and said it was a secret, his voice dropping to that whisper that made Aaliyah's stomach twist into knots. He warned that telling would make Aaliyah's mom sad and break up the family—and Aaliyah loved their mom too much to risk her happiness.

Aaliyah's heart would race every time Chris's car pulled into the driveway. The engine sound that once meant fun now meant danger. They wanted to scream or run away, but their body would just freeze, muscles locking up like someone had poured cement into their veins. They couldn't make themselves say no, couldn't make their voice work, couldn't make their legs move. Afterward, Aaliyah would hide in their room feeling sick and ashamed, curled up under blankets that couldn't make them feel warm or clean, somehow convinced they were the bad one for "letting" it happen.

Now, at 14, Aaliyah feels like they don't fit anywhere. The hallways at school feel too bright, too loud, full of kids who seem to move through life with an ease that Aaliyah can't remember ever feeling. They shrink away from friends who try to include them, worried that people can somehow see their secret written across their face like invisible ink that everyone but Aaliyah can read. They stopped raising their hand in class even though they're smart and used to love the feeling of knowing the right answer—now they feel like they don't deserve attention, don't deserve to take up space. At night, they lie awake replaying those memories like a movie they can't turn off, wondering why they couldn't stop Chris, wondering what they did wrong.

The shame feels like it's suffocating them, wrapping around their chest like a heavy blanket they can't throw off.

Rachel's Story

Rachel's 15 now, but her story started when she was 14 and dating Josh, a junior with confident smile and the kind of easy charm that made adults trust him immediately. He seemed sweet at first—walking her to class, remembering little details about her day, making her feel special and chosen in a way that was intoxicating for someone still figuring out who they were.

But then he started pushing her to do things she wasn't ready for, his requests growing more insistent, his touch lingering in ways that made her uncomfortable. When she'd say no, her voice small but clear, he'd shift tactics, making her feel guilty with words that wrapped around her conscience like thorns: "If you really loved me, you'd do this." "Don't you trust me?" "I thought you were different from other girls." "Everyone else our age is doing this—what's wrong with you?"

Rachel felt trapped in a web she couldn't see clearly. She eventually gave in, but afterward felt horrible—like she'd betrayed some essential part of herself, like she'd handed over something precious and received nothing but emptiness in return. Josh would act like it was no big deal, whistling as he drove her home, chatting about weekend plans as if nothing had changed. This made her feel even worse, like she was being dramatic for nothing, like her feelings didn't matter.

She didn't tell anyone. The thought of explaining to her friends felt impossible—they all thought Josh was perfect, the kind of boyfriend they wished they had. She was scared they would judge her, or worse, not believe her. Her parents would definitely blame her if they found out, she was sure of it.

At school, Rachel started feeling like everyone could tell something was different about her, like shame was a smell clinging to her clothes that she couldn't wash out. She stopped wearing the clothes she liked—the colorful dresses and fitted jeans that used to make her feel confident—worried they made her look like she was "asking for it." When Jake would text her, her phone buzzing with his name, she'd feel physically sick but pretend everything was fine, responding with happy emojis that felt like lies.

The shame made her feel like she was carrying this huge secret that separated her from everyone else, like there was now a glass wall between her and the rest of the world.

Maybe Aaliyah's or Rachel's stories sound familiar. Maybe you feel like you're carrying something that makes you "different" or "less than" other people. But just like with them, that shame came from what someone else did to you—not from anything you did wrong.

The "Name It to Tame It" Principle

Dr. Dan Siegel coined this phrase, and it's particularly powerful with shame. When we name what we're experiencing—"This is shame" rather than "I am bad"—we create distance between ourselves and the feeling.

Naming shame reduces its power, and helps you recognize it as a feeling rather than a fact. It allows you to respond rather than react, and it begins to separate your identity from your experience.

Try it: Next time shame floods you, say (out loud if possible): "I'm experiencing shame right now. This is a feeling, not the truth about me."

A Note About "Parts"

As you read through this book, you'll encounter different "parts" of yourself—the part that froze, the shamed part, the people-pleasing part, and others. This isn't about having multiple personalities. It's about recognizing that trauma creates different aspects of yourself, each with protective roles.

Think of parts like members of a family living in the same house. Sometimes they work together harmoniously, sometimes they conflict. Healing isn't about eliminating parts but helping them communicate and work as a team.

When you encounter exercises asking you to "dialogue with a part," you're not talking to someone else—you're having a conversation between your adult self and these protective aspects. This helps you understand their needs and update their roles for your current, safer life.

Don't worry if this feels strange at first. Parts work is a gentle, effective way to heal trauma without re-traumatizing yourself.

Shame as a Young Part

The voice of shame often isn't your adult self speaking. It's a younger part of you, stuck at the age when the abuse happened. This part absorbed the messages from that time and has been repeating them ever since, searching for logic in chaos.

When shame floods you, you might be hearing from the child part who believed "I must be bad for this to happen," the teenage part who thought "I should have known better," or the part that took on the abuser's voice to feel you had some control.

Dialogue with Your Shamed Part: Next time shame arises, try this. Notice the shame and pause. Ask: "How old is the part of me that feels this shame?" Imagine yourself at that age. What does this younger part need to hear? Let your adult self speak to this part with compassion.

Remember: The shamed part isn't the real you—it's a younger you who needs updating. You can tell this part: "That wasn't our fault. We were just children. We're safe now, and I'm here to protect us."

Common Shame Triggers After Sexual Abuse

Understanding your triggers helps you prepare for and manage shame attacks. Common triggers include sexual situations or discussions, medical exams (especially gynecological/urological), being touched unexpectedly, certain smells, sounds, or places, intimacy or vulnerability, success or happiness (feeling undeserving), making mistakes (proves you're "bad"), someone being kind to you.

When triggered, shame might feel like heat flooding your face, wanting to disappear, your stomach dropping, your chest tightening, an overwhelming urge to hide, or feeling suddenly "dirty" or "wrong."

The Lies Shame Tells (And the Truth That Counters Them)

Shame gets stronger when you hear certain lies—either from other people or from that mean voice in your own head. These myths try to make you think the abuse was somehow your fault. Here are some of the most common ones, and why they're completely wrong.

Shame says: "You're contaminated/dirty/ruined." **Truth:** You're a whole person who survived a terrible experience. Nothing can contaminate your innate worth.

Shame says: "If people knew, they'd reject you." **Truth:** The right people will honor your survival and see your strength. Those who judge weren't safe anyway.

Shame says: "You participated/wanted it/didn't fight hard enough." **Truth:** Survival responses aren't consent. Your body did what it needed to survive. Freezing up is a totally normal way your body responds to danger. It doesn't mean you wanted it or agreed to it.

Shame says: "You're fundamentally different from 'normal' people." **Truth:** You're human. One in three girls and one in five boys experience sexual abuse. You're not alone or abnormal.

Shame says: "You don't deserve good things." **Truth:** You deserve love, respect, safety, and joy—just like every human being.

Additional lies people might tell you include "You must have asked for it." **Truth**: nobody asks to be abused—ever. "You were dressed a certain way, so what did you expect?" **Truth:** your clothes don't cause abuse—abusers do. "Boys can't be victims." anyone can be abused, regardless of gender, and "It wasn't that bad—just get over it." **Truth:** abuse is serious, period.

People who hurt others love these lies because it helps them avoid facing what they've done. Sometimes other people repeat these lies because it's easier than admitting that terrible things can happen to good people, even young people.

But you don't have to carry these lies. They were never yours to begin with.

What actually happened: Someone chose to hurt you. That's not your fault. It doesn't define you. It doesn't make you dirty or broken. You didn't deserve it. You didn't cause it. The fact that you survived is proof of how strong you are, not something to be ashamed of.

Try keeping this truth somewhere you can see it—in your phone, in a notebook, wherever you can see it often: *It is not my fault. I did not deserve it. I am not broken. I can heal.*

When Shame Becomes Self-Harm

Sometimes shame feels so unbearable that hurting yourself seems like the only relief. If you've turned to cutting or other physical self-harm, risky sexual behavior, substance abuse, eating disorders, or severe self-neglect, know this: these aren't signs you're "crazy" or "bad." They're desperate attempts to manage unbearable feelings. It means you've found a way—even though it's not safe—to cope with feelings that feel too big to handle alone.

Trauma can make emotions feel overwhelming, and self-harm might be your body's way of trying to feel calm or numb when the shame and pain take over. That relief you feel afterward is real, but it doesn't last long, and usually the hurt comes back even stronger.

When you were little, you might have needed comfort but learned to keep everything inside, so asking for help feels scary now. You're not weak for trying to handle things yourself—when people let you down, it makes sense to pull away. But your body isn't your enemy. Other people failed you, not your body. You deserve to treat yourself like someone worth caring for.

For now, if shame makes you want to hurt yourself, try these immediate alternatives: hold ice cubes tightly in your hand, snap a rubber band gently on your wrist, draw red lines with a marker where you want to cut, punch a pillow instead of yourself, write down what you want to do then tear it up, try breathing slowly (in for 4 counts, out for 6), do intense exercise, scream into a pillow, tear up paper, or text a crisis line even if you're not sure what to say.

It won't feel perfect at first. It might not feel as intense as what you've done before. But every safe choice is proof that you're learning to take care of the hurt parts of yourself instead of just surviving them.

If self-harm feels like too much to handle, the National Sexual Assault Hotline (1-800-656-HOPE or text RAINN to 741741) can help. But these tools are yours to try right now.

Beginning to Release Shame: The RAIN Technique

Developed by Tara Brach, RAIN is a powerful tool for working with shame:

Example: Recognize: "Shame is here." Allow: "It's okay to feel this." Investigate: "My chest is tight, I want to hide." Nurture: "You're safe now. You survived something terrible. You deserve kindness."

R - Recognize: "I'm feeling shame right now"

A - Allow: Let it be there without fighting it

I - Investigate: Where do I feel this in my body? What does it need?

N - Nurture: Offer yourself compassion, like you would a friend

Practical Shame-Releasing Exercises

The Shame Posture Exercise: Notice how shame makes you want to collapse forward. Gently allow this posture (just slightly). Then slowly straighten, opening your chest. Feel the shift from contraction to expansion. Repeat 2-3 times, noticing the difference.

Write and Burn: Write your shameful thoughts on paper. Read them as if a friend wrote them. Write a compassionate response. Safely burn or tear up the shame thoughts. Keep the compassionate response.

Mirror Work: Start small by looking at your face in the mirror for 10 seconds. Say one kind thing (even "You survived"). Build up slowly and stay for longer times as you can. Notice shame's voice and counter it with truth.

The 5-4-3-2-1 Ground: When shame overwhelms, name 5 things you see, 4 things you can touch, 3 things you hear, 2 things you smell, and 1 thing you taste. This brings you to the present, where you're safe.

Simple Breathing Exercise: When shame feels heavy in your body, place one hand on your heart and one on your belly. Breathe deeply and imagine the shame as a dark cloud inside you. With each exhale, imagine breathing out small pieces of that cloud. You don't have to get rid of it all at once—just letting a little bit go can help.

How to Start Letting Go of Shame

You don't have to stay stuck in shame, even if you're not ready to tell anyone or go to therapy. Healing starts with small, brave steps you can take by yourself.

Call out the shame: Shame gets stronger when you keep it secret, so naming it can make it weaker. Try writing in a journal: "I feel ashamed because of what happened, but it wasn't my fault." You don't have to believe it completely yet—just writing it down helps.

Fight back against the lies: When shame tells you you're "bad" or "unlovable," write down one thing you actually like about yourself. Maybe you're good at listening, or you make people laugh, or you're creative. If that feels too hard, start really small: "I got through today" or "I was kind to my pet."

Help your body feel safe: Shame can make your whole body feel tense and wrong. Try this: sit quietly, take five slow breaths (breathe in for 4 seconds, hold for 4 seconds, breathe out for 4 seconds), and notice how your feet feel on the floor. This helps remind your body that you're safe right now.

Express yourself safely: If talking feels too scary, try drawing, writing poetry, or listening to music that feels like it gets you. You don't have to show anyone—this is just for you.

Imagine a kind voice: Shame sounds like a really mean voice in your head. Try imagining someone kind—maybe a favorite teacher, a friend, or even a character from a show you like—saying things like "You didn't deserve that" or "You're enough just as you are." This can help you start seeing yourself differently.

Remember you're not alone: Shame wants you to feel like you're the only one, but you're not. One in three girls and one in six boys experience sexual abuse, and many of them feel the same shame you do. Reading stories like Aaliyah's or Rachel's can remind you that other people understand what you're going through.

If you ever feel ready to talk to someone, that hotline I mentioned (1-800-656-HOPE or text RAINN to 741741) lets you share without giving your name, and you can hang up anytime. But for now, these small steps can help you start loosening shame's grip on your life.

Creating a Shame-Resilient Life

Releasing shame isn't a one-time event—it's an ongoing practice.

Build Shame Resilience: Practice self-compassion daily, challenge shame thoughts with truth, connect with safe people (even one), share your story when ready (even with yourself), and celebrate small victories over shame.

Create New Neural Pathways: Every time you speak kindly to yourself, recognize shame as a lie, practice the exercises in this book, or choose self-care over self-harm, you're literally rewiring your brain for self-compassion instead of shame.

The Path Forward

Shame thrives in silence, isolation, and judgment. It dies in the presence of truth-telling (even to yourself), self-compassion, safe connection, body-based healing, and patient, persistent practice. You don't have to be shame-free to start healing. You just have to be willing to question shame's lies, one thought at a time.

Why This All Matters

Shame might feel like it's part of who you are, but it's not. It's a lie someone told you when they hurt you, and it's been made worse by a world that sometimes blames survivors instead of the people who actually caused the harm. Understanding how shame works and why it's there can help you start letting it go. Healing from shame is about rediscovering that you're worth something and reconnecting with the world around you. You deserve that.

One Last Thing

You are not defined by what happened to you or the shame you're carrying right now. You're defined by your strength, your heart, and the fact that you're here reading this, trying to understand and heal. Shame might feel incredibly heavy right now, but it doesn't have to stay that way. Every time you choose to be kind to yourself—whether that's writing in a journal, taking a deep breath, or trying a safer way to cope when things get overwhelming—you're pushing shame away and getting a little more of yourself back. *You're not alone in this, and you're stronger than you know.* Keep going, one step at a time.

Coaching Corner: "The Truth About Your Worth"

I want you to know something that took me years to learn: Your worth was never on the table. What happened to you didn't diminish it, can't destroy it, and will never define it. You were born worthy, you remained worthy through everything that happened, and you're worthy right now as you read this. Not because of what you do or don't do, but simply because you exist. That's not something anyone can take from you—not even the person who hurt you.

The shame you feel is not who you are. It's something that attached itself to you during trauma, like smoke clinging to clothes after a fire.

You are not dirty. You are not damaged. You are not less than. You are not defined by what someone did to you.

The shame you carry belongs to the person who chose to hurt you. They should feel ashamed of their actions. You? You should feel proud that you survived, that you're seeking healing, that you're brave enough to read these words.

Here's what I know: shame cannot survive being seen with compassion. Every time you name it ("That's shame talking"), every time you counter its lies with truth, every time you treat yourself with kindness instead of criticism—you're winning.

Take a moment right now. Put your hand on your heart and say: "The shame I feel is not who I am. I am worthy of love and respect, exactly as I am."

That's not just a nice thought. That's the truth shame never wanted you to discover.

6

Coping with Big Feelings: Understanding Self-Harm and Other Responses

Your coping mechanisms were brilliant survival strategies.
Now it's time to update them for a safer world.

WHEN THE PAIN FROM sexual abuse feels too big to hold, you'll do anything—anything—to make it stop, even for just a moment. Maybe you've hurt yourself on purpose. Maybe you've lost yourself in hookups that left you feeling empty. Maybe you've used substances to numb out, or restricted food to feel in control, or taken risks that could destroy you.

If you recognize yourself here, I need you to know: these behaviors don't make you weak, crazy, or bad. They make you human, trying to survive pain that feels un-survivable. There's a massive difference between wanting to die and desperately wanting the pain to stop living in you.

Understanding Your Coping Responses

When trauma from sexual abuse floods your system with unbearable feelings—shame that burns, fear that freezes, rage with nowhere to go, grief that threatens to drown you—your brain scrambles for relief. ANY relief. Even if that relief hurts you more in the long run.

Think of it this way: if you were on fire, you'd jump into any water available, even if it was freezing or polluted. The immediate need to stop burning overrides everything else. That's what trauma coping looks like—desperate attempts to stop the emotional fire, regardless of the consequences.

These coping mechanisms are actually evidence of your will to survive, not signs of weakness. They're your psyche's attempt to make emotional pain physical and therefore more manageable. They create a sense of control when you feel powerless.They numb overwhelming feelings, punish yourself for shame that isn't yours, feel something when you're numb, feel nothing when emotions are too much, and express pain that has no words.

The Hidden Logic of Harmful Coping

Each harmful coping mechanism has its own logic that makes perfect sense in the context of trauma.

Self-Harm (Cutting, Burning, Hitting) converts emotional pain to physical pain which feels more controllable, releases endorphins that temporarily soothe, creates visible evidence of invisible wounds, provides a sense of control, breaks through numbness, and punishes the "bad" self that shame created.

Sexual Self-Harm (Risky Sex, Recreating Abuse) attempts to reclaim control over what was taken, recreates familiar patterns through trauma repetition, confirms beliefs about worth ("I'm only good for this"), provides temporary connection or validation, numbs through intensity, and self-punishes through degradation.

Substance Use numbs unbearable feelings, provides escape from memories, helps you feel "normal," manages anxiety and hypervigilance, enables sleep despite nightmares, and creates artificial calm.

Disordered Eating controls something when everything feels chaotic, makes you smaller or invisible for protection, punishes the body that "betrayed" you, provides structure and rules, numbs through hunger or fullness, and creates a problem you can "solve."

Risk-Taking Behaviors prove you're still alive, provide adrenaline rush that overrides pain, tempt fate when you're ambivalent about living, recreate familiar danger, and distract from internal pain.

Meeting Your Watchdog Parts

When you self-harm, use substances, or engage in risky behaviors, it's often a "watchdog part" desperately trying to alert you to emotional danger or provide relief. These parts learned that when emotional pain gets too big, drastic action is needed.

Think of these watchdog parts like smoke alarms that are too sensitive—they're trying to keep you safe, but they're using outdated or harmful methods. They might include the Cutter ("Physical pain is easier than emotional pain"), the Number ("If I can't feel anything, I can't be hurt"), the Risk-Taker ("At least this makes me feel alive"), or the Escape Artist ("We need to get out of this body NOW").

These aren't bad parts—they're overwhelmed protectors using the only tools they learned.

Updating Your Watchdog Parts: When urges arise, pause and say "I hear you, watchdog. What danger are you sensing?" Thank this part: "Thank you for trying to protect me." Update this part: "We have new tools now. We're learning safer ways." Offer alternatives: "Let's try ice cubes, movement, or calling someone first."

Marcus's Story: When Pain Seeks Release

Marcus was sexually abused by his older cousin from ages 8 to 11 during family gatherings that were supposed to be safe and happy. The abuse happened in a basement rec room that smelled like old carpet and Pine-Sol, while upstairs the adults laughed over card games and the television droned with whatever sports game was on. By 16, he'd never told anyone, and the secret was eating him alive like acid in his chest.

The shame and rage had nowhere to go—until he discovered that hooking up with strangers he met online made him feel powerful for a moment. In control. Like he was finally choosing what happened to his body instead of having it chosen for him. In those brief encounters in empty parking lots or strangers' apartments that smelled like cigarettes and desperation, he felt like he had agency for the first time since he was eight years old.

But afterward, the shame would crash over him even stronger than before, a wave of self-disgust so intense it took his breath away. So he'd drink to numb it, cheap vodka that burned going down and made everything blurry around the edges. When that stopped working, when the alcohol just made him sick without providing relief, he started cutting—small, precise lines on his thighs where no one would see, hidden beneath jeans and long shorts even in summer. The physical pain felt clean, manageable, nothing like the messy chaos raging inside his head.

Marcus wasn't trying to die. He was trying to survive feelings that threatened to tear him apart from the inside out. Each behavior made sense as a survival strategy: the hookups were attempting to reclaim power, the drinking was numbing unbearable shame, and the cutting was making internal pain external and manageable.

Understanding this logic was the first step in Marcus finding healthier ways to cope with the aftermath of what his cousin had stolen from him.

Recognizing Your Patterns

Take a moment to consider your own coping patterns without judgment. When emotions overwhelm you, do you hurt yourself physically, seek intense experiences, sexual or otherwise? Do you use substances to escape, control food or eating, take dangerous risks, or completely shut down and dissociate?

What triggers these urges? It might be specific memories, shame spirals, feeling trapped or powerless, being alone, intimate situations, or stress and conflict.

What are you seeking? Perhaps relief from pain, a sense of control, punishment for perceived "badness," to feel something or anything, to feel nothing, or evidence you're alive.

Understanding your patterns isn't about judgment—it's about recognizing the brilliant , even if harmful, logic of your survival system.

The Bridge: From Harmful to Healing

You don't have to stop harmful coping cold turkey (and for some things, like substances, that could be dangerous). Instead, think of building a bridge—adding safer options while you still have access to old patterns if absolutely needed.

Harm Reduction Approach: If you're going to cut, use clean tools and care for wounds. If you're having risky sex, use protection and choose safer partners. If you're using substances, don't use alone and test what you're taking. If you're restricting food, add one safe food. If you're taking risks, wear a helmet or seatbelt.

This isn't endorsing harmful behaviors—it's acknowledging that shame and perfectionism don't help. Safety first, always.

Safer Alternatives That Actually Work

These alternatives work because they provide similar relief without the lasting harm.

Instead of Cutting/Physical Self-Harm: Try ice cubes (hold them tight or run them over skin for intense sensation without damage), rubber band (snap on wrist for sharp sensation), red marker (draw on skin where you want to cut for visual without wound), exercise (intense workout until exhaustion for physical release), cold shower (shock to system that's completely safe), or scream therapy (into pillow or in car for emotional release).

Instead of Sexual Self-Harm: Try self-massage (reclaim safe, caring touch), dance (move your body for yourself), create boundaries list (what you will and won't accept), write about healthy intimacy (what it would look like), practice saying no (to small things first), or connect non-sexually (focus on friendships).

Instead of Numbing Out: Try breathing exercises (4-7-8 breath for calm, inhale 4, hold 7, exhale 8)), meditation apps (guided practices for anxiety), bilateral stimulation (cross-lateral movements), grounding exercises (5-4-3-2-1 sensory), creative expression (art, music, writing), or safe spaces (blanket fort, bath, nature).

When You Need Control: Try organizing something (drawer, playlist, photos), create art (you control every element), exercise routine (structured, measurable progress), learn something new (skill you can master), garden (nurture and control growth), or cook and bake (follow or modify recipes).

The "Riding the Wave" Technique

Urges to self-harm are like waves—they build, crest, and eventually subside. Most urges peak within 20-30 minutes. Your job isn't to stop the wave but to surf it safely.

Notice: "I'm having an urge to [behavior]." Breathe: Deep belly breaths to stay present. Set a timer: 20 minutes before acting. Distract: Use alternative coping for those 20 minutes. Check in: How strong is the urge now? Repeat if needed. Urges will pass in just a bit.

Remember: You're not trying to never have urges. You're learning to respond differently when they arise.

Creating Your Safety Plan

Before crisis hits, create your plan.

My Warning Signs:

Physical sensations that signal distress:

_____

_____

Thoughts that spiral toward self-harm:

_____

_____

Situations that trigger urges:

_____

_____

My Alternatives:

3 physical alternatives (ice, exercise, etc.)

_____   _____   _____

3 soothing alternatives (bath, music, etc.)

_____   _____   _____

3 connection alternatives (text friend, hotline, etc.)

_____   _____   _____

My Support Network:

Crisis line numbers (988, RAINN: 1-800-656-4673),

Safe friend number _____

Therapist/counselor contact _____

My Reasons to Stay Safe:

However small (my pet needs me, I am curious about tomorrow, spite)

_____ _____ _____

Future goals (however distant)

_____ _____ _____

People who'd miss me (however few)

_____ _____ _____

The Long Road to Different Coping

Changing coping mechanisms is like learning a new language. At first, the old patterns feel natural and the new ones feel forced. But with practice, new responses become more automatic, urges become less intense, you develop preference for safer coping, self-compassion replaces self-punishment, and life becomes more livable.

This isn't about perfection. You might return to old patterns during extreme stress. That's not failure—it's human. What matters is the overall trajectory toward safer, kinder ways of surviving.

> **Coaching Corner: "Your Pain Deserves Compassionate Response"**
>
> Every time you've hurt yourself, you were trying to survive overwhelming pain. Every. Single. Time. You weren't being "dramatic" or "attention-seeking" or "weak." You were drowning and grabbing the only life preserver you could find, even if it had holes in it.
>
> Now you're learning that there are better life preservers available. Ones that won't hurt you more. Ones that honor your pain without adding to it.
>
> This transition is hard. The old ways are familiar, immediately effective, and strangely comforting. The new ways feel uncertain, slower to work, and require faith they'll help. Be patient with yourself.
>
> You learned *harmful coping* to survive trauma you didn't choose. You can learn *healing coping* to build a life you do choose. Not because you "should" or because others want you to, but because you deserve responses to your pain that don't create more pain.
>
> Your wounds deserve tender care, not more wounding. Your pain deserves acknowledgment, not punishment. You deserve coping that helps you heal, not just survive.
>
> One safer choice at a time. One wave ridden without drowning. One moment of self-compassion instead of self-harm. That's how you build a different future—brave moment by brave moment.

7

How Trauma Shows Up: Recognizing Your Symptoms

The body keeps the score, but you get to rewrite the game.

H AVE YOU EVER FELT like something's wrong with you but you can't put your finger on what? Like you're constantly anxious for "no reason," or you snap at people you care about, or you can't sleep even though you're exhausted?

Maybe you've been telling yourself you're just stressed about work, or you're naturally moody, or you're being dramatic. But what if I told you these might actually be signs that your mind and body are still processing something that happened to you?

This chapter is about recognizing how trauma from sexual abuse can show up in your daily life—sometimes in ways that seem totally unrelated to what happened. Understanding these symptoms isn't about labeling yourself or making excuses. It's about finally making sense of what you've been feeling and knowing that you're not crazy, you're not broken, and you're definitely not alone.

Why Trauma Symptoms Feel So Random

Here's the thing about trauma: it doesn't follow rules. It doesn't show up the way you'd expect. You might think that if something bad happened to you, you'd just feel sad about that specific thing. But trauma is sneakier than that.

Your brain's number one job is keeping you safe. When you experience sexual abuse, your brain goes into overdrive trying to protect you from ever being hurt like that again. It starts seeing danger everywhere. It keeps you on high alert. It might even make you disconnect from your feelings entirely because feeling is too risky.

These protective mechanisms were brilliant in the moment—they helped you survive. But now they might be making your daily life really hard. And trauma can affect how you navigate relationships, how you connect with others, and how you see yourself, regardless of when it happened in your life.

The symptoms you're experiencing aren't signs of weakness. They're evidence that your brain is doing exactly what brains do: trying to keep you safe based on what it learned from a dangerous situation.

Kia's Story: When Everything Feels Wrong

Let me share Kia's story, which shows how trauma symptoms can affect every part of your life.

When Kia was 12, her soccer coach—someone everyone loved and trusted—started giving her "special attention." The man had kind eyes that crinkled when he smiled at parents during games, and his voice carried easily across the field with encouraging shouts. But during those extra practice sessions, when the afternoon sun cast long shadows across the empty field and the air still smelled of fresh-cut grass, everything changed.

The coach would touch Kia inappropriately, always acting like it was normal, part of making Kia a better player. His hands felt too warm through her jersey, and she could smell his sharp aftershave mixing with sweat. Kia froze every time, her cleats seeming to grow roots into the ground, confused and scared, not understanding why her body wouldn't move or why her voice disappeared when she needed it most.

By the time Kia turned 23, she felt like a completely different person from that confident girl who used to race down the field. She was constantly on edge, her shoulders permanently hunched as if bracing for impact, her body tense like she was ready to run at any moment. Little things would set her off—a colleague's hand on her shoulder would make her flinch so hard she knocked over her coffee, certain cologne scents in elevators would make her feel sick and dizzy, and she'd snap at her roommate over nothing, leaving them confused and hurt.

Sleep became her enemy. She'd lie awake for hours listening to every creak of her apartment building, every car passing on the street outside. When she finally drifted off, nightmares would jolt her awake, her sheets soaked with sweat and her heart pounding so hard she was sure her neighbors could hear it through the walls. She started getting headaches that felt like someone was tightening a vise around her skull. Her stomach hurt so often—a constant churning that made her push food around her plate—that her worried friends suggested she see doctor after doctor, but no one found anything wrong.

Kia avoided sports entirely, telling everyone she was "over that phase," but really she couldn't stand being in gyms where the smell of rubber mats and cleaning supplies brought back flashes of those after-practice moments. She pulled away from dating, creating excuses whenever potential partners wanted to get closer. She couldn't explain why intimacy felt so hard now, why she always needed to know where the exits were, why she always felt like she had to watch her back.

The worst part? Kia didn't connect any of this to what her coach did. She just thought she was messed up, weak, going crazy. It wasn't until a therapist mentioned that stress can cause physical symptoms that Kia started wondering if maybe her body was trying to tell her something.

When Kia began journaling—just writing down what she felt without trying to fix it—patterns emerged. She noticed she felt worst on Tuesdays, which had been her old practice days. Her headaches came when she smelled that specific deodorant her coach used, now recognizing it on other men in stores and offices. Understanding these connections didn't magically fix everything, but it helped Kia realize she wasn't losing her mind. Her body and brain were responding to trauma in the only way they knew how.

The Many Faces of Trauma Symptoms

Trauma symptoms can show up in every part of your life. Here's what survivors commonly experience:

Physical symptoms often manifest as feeling jumpy, tense, or constantly "on edge," along with exhaustion that sleep doesn't seem to fix. Many people experience unexplained headaches, stomachaches, or pain with no clear medical cause, plus trouble falling asleep, staying asleep, or having nightmares. You might notice your heart racing or trouble breathing that seems to come "out of nowhere," feeling numb or disconnected from your body, or becoming super sensitive to certain smells, sounds, or sensations.

Mental and cognitive effects typically include anxiety that feels constant or comes in overwhelming waves, along with intrusive thoughts or memories you can't shake. Many people describe feeling spacey, foggy, or like they're watching life from outside themselves. Trouble concentrating or remembering things is common, as are feelings of worthlessness, shame, or being fundamentally different from others. Depression often feels heavy and endless, sometimes accompanied by thoughts of escaping or not wanting to exist.

Emotional patterns frequently involve anger that explodes seemingly out of nowhere, sadness that doesn't match current circumstances, or feeling emotionally numb when you think you "should" feel something. Persistent guilt or shame, fear that doesn't make logical sense, and mood swings that feel completely out of control are also common experiences.

Relationship challenges often include difficulty trusting anyone, even people who've never hurt you, plus feeling uncomfortable with physical closeness or intimacy. You might find yourself pushing people away when they try to help, feeling like no one could understand if you told them what happened, swinging between being overly clingy or completely distant, and struggling with setting boundaries or saying no.

Daily life disruptions can involve avoiding places, people, or things that remind you of what happened, using alcohol, drugs, or other escapes to cope, or developing perfectionism where you feel you have to be "good" all the time. Some people engage in risky behaviors that could cause harm, experience trouble with school, work focus, or motivation, and notice significant changes in their eating, sleeping, or self-care routines.

Remember: having some of these symptoms doesn't mean you're damaged. It means you're human and you've been through something hard.

Simple Ways to Track What You're Feeling

You don't need to analyze everything or have it all figured out. Sometimes just noticing is enough. Here are some low-key ways to start recognizing your symptoms:

The Daily Check-In: Once a day, ask yourself: "What's one thing I noticed about how I felt today?" Write it down or just think about it. No judgment, just noticing.

The Pattern Spotter: Keep a simple note in your phone. When something feels really hard, jot down what happened, how you felt, and what time or day it was. After a few weeks, look for patterns.

The Body Scan: Before bed, do a quick mental scan from head to toe. Where do you hold tension? What hurts? What feels okay? Just notice without trying to fix anything.

The Trigger Map: Make a list of things that make you feel suddenly awful—certain smells, sounds, or sights; specific situations or places;

types of touch or closeness. This helps you understand what your brain associates with danger.

The Good Moments List: Also track when you feel okay or even good. What helps? What makes you feel safer? This is just as important as noticing the hard stuff.

What To Do With What You Notice

Recognizing symptoms is powerful, but it's just the first step. Here's what you can do with this awareness:

Validate yourself: "Of course I feel this way. I've been through something hard."

Get curious, not critical: "I wonder why Tuesdays are hard" instead of "I'm so stupid for feeling this way." Be curious about your symptoms. Like a scientist collecting data. Not to judge it, just curious about the information.

Make small adjustments: If you know crowds make you anxious, can you stand near exits? If certain smells trigger you, can you carry something that smells safe?

Use your coping tools: When you notice symptoms arising, try the breathing exercises, grounding techniques, or safe coping strategies from other chapters.

Remember it's temporary: Symptoms feel permanent but they're not. They can and do get better.

Somatic Exercise for Calming Your Nervous System: When you notice anxiety or tension building, try this: Place both hands on your chest, one over the other. Press gently and take three deep breaths, feeling your chest rise and fall under your hands. This simple pressure and awareness can help signal safety to your nervous system.

Why Recognition Matters

Here's why taking time to recognize your symptoms is so important:

You're not crazy: Understanding that these are trauma symptoms, not character flaws, can be incredibly relieving.

You can predict and prepare: If you know what triggers you, you can plan ahead and feel more in control.

You can communicate better: Even if you're not ready to share your trauma, you can say things like "I get anxious in crowds" or "I need space when I'm upset."

You can track progress: Noticing symptoms also means noticing when they get better, even a little bit.

You can be gentler with yourself: Instead of getting mad at yourself for being "weak," you can recognize you're dealing with legitimate trauma responses.

The Truth About Your Symptoms

Your symptoms are not your fault. They're not signs that you're weak, dramatic, or broken. They're evidence that you survived something difficult and your brain and body are still working to protect you.

One in three girls and one in six boys experience sexual abuse. Many of them have symptoms just like yours. You're not alone in feeling this way, and you're not alone in the journey toward healing.

Some days will be harder than others. Some symptoms might get worse before they get better. That's normal. Healing isn't a straight line—it's a winding path with setbacks and breakthroughs.

Moving Forward

Every time you notice a symptom without judging yourself, every time you respond to your struggles with compassion instead of criticism, every time you use a healthy coping strategy—you're rewiring your brain. You're teaching it that you're safe now, that you can handle hard feelings, that you're stronger than what happened to you.

You don't have to have it all figured out. You don't have to heal on anyone else's timeline. You just have to keep noticing, keep being gentle with yourself, and keep taking one small step at a time.

Your symptoms don't define you. They're just signals—messages from a brain and body that are trying their best to keep you safe. Listen to them with kindness. Respond to them with care. And remember: *you've already survived the hardest part.* Everything from here is about learning to thrive.

Coaching Corner: Your Symptoms Are Your Strength

Those symptoms you're experiencing? They're not flaws or weaknesses. They're proof that your body and mind did everything possible to protect you. Every symptom is a survival strategy that helped you get through something impossible. Yes, they might not be serving you well anymore, and yes, we want to help them evolve into healthier patterns. But first, can we just acknowledge how incredible it is that you survived? Your symptoms are evidence of your strength, not your brokenness. Honor them, then gently help them transform.

8

Understanding Trauma-Based Behaviors vs. Personality

You are not your coping mechanisms. You are the one who survived.

O NE OF THE MOST healing questions I ever learned to ask wasn't "What's wrong with me?" It was "What happened to me?" That shift—from judgment to curiosity—changed everything.

If you've grown up being labeled as "too sensitive," "dramatic," "cold," "needy," "controlling," "lazy," or "difficult," you might have absorbed those labels as truth about who you are. But what if they're not who you are at all? What if they're just your nervous system's way of saying "I'm still not okay with what happened"?

This chapter is about separating what's truly you from what's actually unhealed trauma. It's about understanding that many of your "personality traits" might actually be brilliant survival strategies that just haven't gotten the memo that you're safer now.

Trauma Is Not Your Identity

Having trauma doesn't mean you're broken. It means you're human and you survived something that no one should have to survive. The coping mechanisms that developed weren't character flaws—they were superpowers that helped you endure the unendurable. But here's the empowering truth: what your nervous system learned, it can un-learn. The adaptations that helped you survive then might be limiting you now, but they can shift. Not through willpower or positive think-ing, but through gentle, body-based practices that teach your nervous system it's safe now.

The Labels That Stick

Think about the words people have used to describe you. Maybe even words you use to describe yourself: "I'm just naturally anxious," "I'm a people pleaser," "I'm bad at relationships," "I'm too emotional," "I'm cold and distant," "I'm a control freak," "I'm oversensitive," or "I'm just not a trusting person."

Now here's the radical thought: What if none of these are fixed person-ality traits? What if they're all adaptive responses to trauma that got stuck in the "on" position?

How Trauma Shapes "Personality"

When trauma happens, especially in childhood or adolescence, our brains and bodies adapt to survive. These adaptations are brilliant in the moment—they keep us as safe as possible in unsafe situations. The problem is, they often outlive their usefulness.

The People Pleaser: What looks like "always putting others first, can't say no, needs everyone to be happy" might actually be a trauma adaptation that learned keeping others happy equals staying safe. Maybe anger in your house was dangerous. Maybe love was conditional on being "good." Your nervous system learned: make everyone happy or bad things happen.

The Overachiever: What appears as "perfectionist, workaholic, never satisfied" might be an adaptation that discovered achieving made you valuable, worthy of protection or praise. Or maybe it was a way to control something when everything else felt chaotic. Your nervous system learned: if I'm perfect, I'm safe.

The Rebel: What seems like "defiant, angry, pushes people away" might be an adaptation that figured out offense is the best defense. If you push people away first, they can't hurt you. If you stay angry, you don't have to feel the vulnerable emotions underneath. Your nervous system learned: connection is dangerous, anger is power.

The Ghost: What looks like "withdrawn, quiet, naturally introverted" might be an adaptation that realized being invisible meant being safe. The smaller you made yourself, the less likely you were to be targeted. Your nervous system learned: being seen equals danger.

The Caretaker: What appears as "always helping others, can't handle being helped" might be an adaptation that found taking care of others gave you purpose, control, or deflected attention from your own pain. Your nervous system learned: my needs don't matter, but I matter if I'm useful.

Kelly's Story: Mistaking Adaptation for Identity

Kelly came to understand this distinction in a powerful way. She'd always thought she was just "too intense" for people. Too emotional. Too much.

She believed that her sensitivity, her tendency to overreact, and her fierce independence were simply her personality—flaws she had to manage. For years, she wore labels like "dramatic," "needy," or "cold," depending on the season of life and who was doing the naming. Teachers called her "too sensitive" when she cried easily. Friends called her "dramatic" when she had big reactions to small slights. Family called her "cold" when she withdrew and stopped sharing her feelings.

But as she began exploring her story in therapy, something powerful emerged. Her so-called "overreactions" weren't random emotional outbursts—they were rooted in early betrayals and boundary violations that had taught her young nervous system that small threats could quickly become big dangers. Her fierce independence wasn't a personality trait—it was a shield she built stone by stone when no one came to protect her, when asking for help had been met with dismissal or worse. Her sensitivity wasn't weakness—it was the finely tuned radar she developed to keep herself safe in environments that weren't, scanning constantly for shifts in mood and tone that might signal incoming harm.

She had mistaken her adaptations for identity, her survival strategies for character flaws.

The truth was: beneath the survival patterns lived someone deeply intuitive, relationally gifted, and wise. She wasn't broken—she had been brilliantly wired for survival in an environment that demanded it. And now, in safety, she was beginning the journey back to her truest self—not by changing who she was, but by understanding why she became that way and choosing consciously which patterns still served her.

The Confusion This Creates

It's disorienting to realize that what you've always thought of as "you" might actually be trauma. Some common thoughts include "But I've always been this way." *Maybe, or maybe you've been this way since the trauma and can't remember before clearly.* "But my family says I'm just..." *Families often mislabel trauma responses, especially if they were part of the traumatic environment.* "But I don't want to blame everything on trauma." *This isn't about blame but understanding, and understanding creates choice.* "If this isn't me, then who am I?" *You are the person underneath the adaptations, waiting to be discovered.*

Behaviors That Confuse Survivors

These trauma adaptations often show up in confusing ways.

Pushing Away What You Want: You crave connection but sabotage relationships. You want success but self-destruct when things go well. This isn't self-sabotage as much as self-protection—your nervous system is trying to keep you from vulnerability.

Emotional Extremes: You're either completely shut down or totally overwhelmed. There's no middle ground because trauma disrupts emotional regulation. This isn't being "dramatic"—it's nervous system dysregulation.

Hypervigilance Disguised as Intuition: You "just know" when something's wrong (because you're constantly scanning for danger). You can't relax (because relaxing once meant missing warning signs). This isn't psychic ability—it's trauma-based hyperawareness.

Relationship Patterns: You attract the same type of harmful people. You can't maintain healthy relationships. You're either completely dependent or totally independent. These aren't character flaws—they're trauma patterns playing out.

The Freedom in Understanding

When you realize that these "personality traits" are actually trauma adaptations, everything changes. You stop judging yourself—instead of "Why am I so needy?" you think "My nervous system is seeking the safety it didn't have." You gain compassion—instead of "I'm so messed up," you think "I adapted brilliantly to survive." You see possibility—instead of "This is just who I am," you think "This is who I became to survive, and I can become something else." You find choice—instead of automatic responses, you start to notice: "Oh, that's my trauma talking. What does the real me want?"

Your Parts Are Not Your Personality

Understanding Your Internal System

What you think of as "personality traits" might actually be parts of you that got stuck in protective roles. After trauma, these parts can become so dominant that you mistake them for who you are. But they're not your identity—they're your survival team.

Common Parts Mistaken for Personality

"I'm just a people pleaser" is actually a protective part that learned safety comes from keeping others happy. What this part needs: to know that disappointing others won't lead to abuse.

"I'm naturally anxious" is actually a hypervigilant part still scanning for danger. What this part needs: regular reminders that the danger has passed.

"I'm cold and distant" is actually a protective part that uses walls to prevent future hurt. What this part needs: to learn that some people can be trusted.

"I'm a control freak" is actually a part trying to prevent chaos and unpredictability. What this part needs: to experience safety even when not in control.

"I'm too sensitive" is actually a part with finely-tuned danger detection. What this part needs: validation that this sensitivity once kept you safe.

Mapping Your Parts System

List your "personality traits" that feel limiting. For each one, ask "What part of me acts this way?" Consider "How old does this part feel?" Explore "What was this part protecting me from?" Thank each part for its service. Let your adult self lead with: "I see you. You helped us survive. Let's update your job description."

Discovering Your True Self

So how do you figure out what's you and what's trauma? Here are some ways to explore:

1. The Before and After: If you can remember life before trauma, what were you like? What did you enjoy? What felt natural? (If trauma started very young, this might not be possible, and that's okay.)

2. The Opposite Experiment: Take a "personality trait" and try its opposite in small, safe ways. Always say yes? Try saying no to something tiny. Always independent? Ask for one small favor. Always serious? Watch something silly. Notice how it feels. Foreign doesn't mean wrong—it might mean new.

3. The Body Check: Your body knows the difference between authentic self and trauma adaptation. True self feels expansive, lighter. Trauma adaptations feel tense, restricted.

4. The Joy Detective: What brings you genuine joy (not just relief or numbness)? Those moments of joy are clues to your true self.

5. The Values Excavation: Under the trauma responses, what do you truly value? Connection? Creativity? Peace? Those values point to who you really are.

> **Somatic Exercise for True Self Discovery:** Stand with your feet hip-width apart. Place one hand on your heart and one on your belly. Breathe deeply and ask yourself, "Who am I beneath all the protection?" Don't force an answer. Just breathe and notice what arises in your body. Sometimes your true self speaks in sensations before words.

Common Trauma Adaptations Mistaken for Personality

"I'm just not a feelings person" might actually be that emotions were dangerous in my environment. "I'm a control freak" might actually be that I need control because I had none when it mattered. "I'm bad at relationships" might actually be that I never learned how safe relationships work. "I'm too sensitive" might actually be that my nervous system is still on high alert. "I'm a pessimist" might actually be that expecting the worst helped me survive. "I'm not creative/smart/capable" might actually be that I learned to hide my gifts to stay safe.

The Integration Process

You don't have to throw out all your adaptations. Some served you well and might still be useful. The goal is choice—knowing what's trauma adaptation and choosing when to use it versus when to try something new.

Keep What Serves You: Maybe hypervigilance helps you in your career. Keep it there, but learn to turn it off at home.

Modify What Partially Works: Maybe people-pleasing helps you connect, but goes too far. Learn to please others AND yourself.

Release What Hurts You: Maybe self-isolation protected you once but now causes pain. Practice tiny connections.

A Deeper Reflection

Sometimes the most profound discoveries come from the simplest questions. Consider Kayla's story:

Kayla always thought she was just "naturally guarded, disconnected, uninterested in deep relationships." She'd built her identity around being the independent one, the one who didn't need anybody, the one who was fine on her own.

For years, she had accepted that she was simply quiet, cautious, and didn't need others. Her family reinforced this, calling her "the strong one" and "self-sufficient," praising her for never being a burden. But when she began working through her trauma story, she started to notice something deeper. Her distance wasn't a personality trait—it was self-protection layered on so thick she'd forgotten there was anything underneath. Her lack of connection wasn't apathy—it was fear of being hurt again, dressed up as preference. Her silence wasn't shyness—it was learned invisibility, perfected over years of practice. Realizing that much of her "personality" was actually layered survival strategies was both painful and freeing. Painful—because she didn't know who she was underneath it all. If independence wasn't her nature but her protection, if strength wasn't her gift but her armor, then who was she really?Freeing—because for the first time, she had a choice. She could keep the parts that served her and question the parts that isolated her.

And as she kept showing up, doing the work, she discovered parts of herself that had been buried for years. She wasn't emotionally detached—she was deeply empathetic, so much so that she'd learned to shut it down to survive. She wasn't cold—she was cautious, which made sense given what she'd survived. She wasn't uninterested in others—she was unsure if they were safe, which was wisdom, not pathology. You might be in that same space right now—unpacking years of adaptations that kept you safe but also kept you hidden from yourself and others. The real you is still in there, waiting to emerge when it's safe. Maybe now is that time. Maybe you're ready to ask gently: "Is this who I truly am—or who I became to survive?"

YOUR BILL OF RIGHTS

YOU HAVE THE RIGHT TO QUESTION EVERY LABEL EVER PUT ON YOU

YOU HAVE THE RIGHT TO DISCOVER WHO YOU ARE BENEATH THE ADAPTATIONS

YOU HAVE THE RIGHT TO KEEP WHAT SERVES YOU AND RELEASE WHAT DOESN'T

YOU HAVE THE RIGHT TO CHANGE EVEN IF OTHERS RESIST

YOU HAVE THE RIGHT TO BE INCONSISTENT AS YOU FIGURE YOURSELF OUT

YOU HAVE THE RIGHT TO GRIEVE WHO YOU MIGHT HAVE BEEN

YOU HAVE THE RIGHT TO CELEBRATE WHO YOU'RE BECOMING

YOU HAVE THE RIGHT TO TAKE AS LONG AS YOU NEED

Moving Forward With Compassion

This process of separating trauma adaptations from true self isn't quick or easy. You might feel like you're losing yourself before you find yourself. That's normal. You're not losing yourself—you're losing the protective shell that kept you safe.

Some days you'll act from trauma. That's okay. Notice it with curiosity, not judgment: "Oh, there's that pattern again. What's it trying to protect me from?"

Some days you'll glimpse your true self. Celebrate those moments, however brief. That's you, peeking through, checking if it's safe to come out more fully.

The Bottom Line

You are not your trauma responses. You are not your coping mechanisms. You are not your survival strategies. You are the consciousness underneath all of that, the one who survived, the one who's reading this and wondering, "Could I be different?"

Yes. You can be different. Not because you're broken and need fixing, but because you're adaptive and can choose new adaptations now that you're safer.

Your trauma shaped you, but it doesn't define you. Your responses saved you, but they don't limit you. Your personality isn't set in stone—it's a living, breathing thing that can grow and change as you heal.

The question isn't "What's wrong with me?" It never was. The question is "What happened to me, and who do I want to become now?"

That's a question worth exploring, with all the patience and compassion you can give yourself. Your true self is under there, waiting to be discovered. They're not broken. They're not wrong. They're just waiting for you to realize it's safe to come home to yourself.

Coaching Corner: The You That's Always Been There

Imagine peeling an onion—layer by layer of adaptations, protections, and survival strategies. At the center isn't emptiness. At the center is the you that's always been there. The you that existed before trauma taught you to hide. The you that will exist after healing shows you it's safe to emerge. That core self isn't damaged by what happened—it's preserved, waiting. Every adaptation you developed was your psyche's way of protecting that true self until it was safe to come out again. That time might be now. Listen closely—can you hear them in there, waiting to be welcomed home?

9

Noticing Thought Patterns: Spotting and Challenging Lies

Your thoughts are not facts. They're just old programming,
and you're the programmer who can rewrite the code.

I F YOU'VE EVER CAUGHT yourself thinking "I'm worthless," "I deserved what happened," or "No one will ever love me if they knew," you're not alone. These thoughts can feel so real, so true, that you might think they're just facts about who you are.

Mind-Body Connection: Negative thoughts often create physical sensations—tension, numbness, or pain. When practicing thought challenging, notice what happens in your body. If you struggle to feel physical sensations, return to the body awareness exercises from Chapter 1.

But here's what I need you to know: they're not facts. They're lies that trauma planted in your mind, often placed there by the person who hurt you or by the shame that followed. I know because I carried these exact thoughts for years after my own abuse. As both a survivor and a life coach, I've learned that these thoughts are just patterns—mental habits that can be changed. This chapter is about learning to catch those lies in action, challenging them with truth, and slowly rewiring your brain to be kinder to yourself.

Understanding Your Thought Patterns and Neuroplasticity

Your brain is constantly trying to make sense of the world, creating stories to explain what happens to you. When you experience something as confusing and painful as sexual abuse, your brain scrambles to create a story that makes sense. Unfortunately, the story it often lands on is: "This must be my fault."

Why? Because believing you had some control over what happened feels safer than accepting that something terrible happened for no reason at all. If it was your fault, your brain reasons, then you can prevent it from happening again by being "better" or "different."

But this protective mechanism becomes a prison. Those thoughts—"I'm dirty," "I'm broken," "I asked for it"—start playing on repeat until they feel like the soundtrack of your life. Trauma literally changes your brain's wiring, creating mental grooves that your thoughts fall into automatically.

Here's the amazing news about your brain: it has something called neuroplasticity. This means your brain can literally rewire itself throughout your entire life. Every thought you think, every new pattern you practice, physically changes the structure of your brain. Scientists used to believe our brains were fixed after childhood, but now we know that's completely wrong. Your brain is constantly changing based on what you practice.

Think of it like this: trauma created highways in your brain for negative thoughts to travel quickly. But every time you challenge those thoughts, every time you choose a different mental path, you're creating new roads. At first, these new paths are like walking through thick forest—difficult and slow. But the more you use them, the clearer and easier they become. Meanwhile, those old trauma highways start to grow over from lack of use.

This isn't just feel-good talk—it's neuroscience. Studies show that practices like challenging negative thoughts, mindfulness, and self-compassion literally change brain structure. The parts of your brain associated with fear and threat detection can calm down. The parts associated with emotional regulation and self-compassion can grow stronger. You're not stuck with the brain trauma gave you. You can build a new one, thought by thought.

Where These Lies Come From

Let's be clear about where these toxic thoughts actually originate:

From the Abuser: They might have said things like: "This is what you wanted." "No one will believe you." "This is our special secret." "You're mature for your age." "If you tell, I'll hurt someone you love."

From Shame: Your brain creates thoughts like: "I should have fought harder." "I must have done something to cause this." "I'm disgusting now." "Real victims would have said no."

From Society: Messages you've absorbed like: "Boys/men can't be victims." "If you didn't fight, it wasn't real abuse." "What were you wearing?" "Why didn't you tell someone sooner?"

When I was abused as a child, I was told that telling would destroy my family. That lie became the thought "I'm responsible for everyone else's happiness." When my boyfriend pressured me at 15, I thought "I must not be good enough if I can't make him respect my boundaries." These weren't my thoughts—they were poison left behind by people who hurt me.

Alejandro's Story: When Lies Feel Like Truth

Let me tell you about Alejandro, whose story shows how these thought patterns take hold and how to fight back.

Alejandro was 9 when his uncle Ben started the "special games." Ben was the family favorite—the uncle who taught the kids card tricks and always brought the best Christmas presents. Everyone loved him.

But when they were alone, Ben would touch Alejandro in ways that made him feel gross. "This is how uncles show love," Ben would say. "But it's our secret because other people wouldn't understand."

Alejandro's body would freeze every time. Afterward, lying in bed staring at his bedroom ceiling with its glow-in-the-dark stars, his eight-year-old mind would desperately try to make sense of what happened: "Uncle Ben is good—everyone says so. Mom trusts him. If something bad happened, it must be because of me. I must have done something wrong. There's something bad inside me that made this happen."

These weren't just passing thoughts. They became the foundation of how Alejandro understood himself. By age ten, when he struggled with math homework, the voice in his head would whisper, "You can't figure this out because you're stupid—just like you're bad." When friends at recess would choose teams and he'd get picked last, that same voice would confirm, "See? They can sense something's wrong with you."

By 14, these beliefs had crystallized into an unshakeable core identity: "I am fundamentally flawed. I am disgusting. I am bad." Every disappointment, every small failure, every moment of social awkwardness became evidence supporting this central lie. Failed a test? "Of course I did—bad people don't deserve to succeed." Friends invite him somewhere? "They wouldn't want me there if they really knew what I am." Missed a goal in soccer? "I ruin everything I touch."

The thoughts felt absolutely true because they'd been growing in his mind for six years, watered by shame and tended by secrecy.

The spark that changed everything came during his freshman health class. Mrs. Rodriguez was teaching about child safety, and she said something that stopped Alejandro cold: "Children are never responsible for what adults do to them. Never. A child's brain isn't developed enough to consent to or cause adult behavior. When something happens to a child, it's always—always—the adult's responsibility."

Alejandro felt something crack open in his chest. For the first time, he heard his eight-year-old logic from the outside: How could a small child cause an adult to do anything? How could an eight-year-old be responsible for an adult's choices?

That night, he started paying attention to the voice in his head differently. When he bombed a history quiz and immediately thought "because I'm worthless," he caught himself and wondered: "Wait—is this my voice, or is this what I learned to think about myself when I was eight years old?"

That's when he began to fight back, one thought at a time, learning to question the voice that sounded like his own but spoke Ben's planted lies.

Common Thought Patterns After Abuse

Here are the most common lies trauma tells, and the truth that counters them:

The Lie: "It was my fault" shows up as "I should have said no louder," "I shouldn't have been there," or "I led them on." The truth is that the only person responsible for abuse is the abuser. Always.

The Lie: "I'm damaged/broken/ruined" shows up as "No one will want me now," "I'm used goods," or "I'll never be normal." The truth is that you're a whole person who experienced something difficult. You're not broken—you're surviving.

The Lie: "I'm worthless" shows up as "I don't deserve good things," "I'm not as good as other people," or "I don't matter." The truth is that your worth isn't determined by what happened to you. You matter simply because you exist.

The Lie: "I can't trust anyone" shows up as "Everyone will hurt me," "People are dangerous," or "I'm better off alone." The truth is that the person who hurt you doesn't represent everyone. Safe people exist.

The Lie: "I'm dirty/disgusting" shows up as physical discomfort with your body, obsessive washing, or avoiding mirrors. The truth is that nothing that happened to you changed your inherent goodness or cleanliness.

Tools to Spot and Challenge These Lies

Here's your toolkit for catching these thoughts and fighting back:

1. The Thought Catch When you notice yourself feeling bad, pause and ask: "What thought just went through my head?" Write it down exactly as it appeared. Don't judge it, just catch it like you're taking a photograph.

2. The Source Check Ask yourself: "Where did I learn this thought?" Can you trace it back to something the abuser said or implied, a fear they created, or a message from someone who doesn't understand trauma? Recognizing the source helps you see the thought as something given to you, not something true about you.

3. The Evidence Test Like a detective, look for actual evidence. If the thought is "I'm worthless," what evidence supports that? What evidence contradicts it? List real examples: times you've helped someone, things you're good at, people who care about you. Notice how the evidence against the lie is usually stronger.

4. The Friend Test Ask yourself: "If my best friend told me this happened to them, would I think these thoughts about them?" Would you tell your friend they're dirty, broken, or at fault? Of course not. You deserve the same compassion you'd give others.

5. The Rewrite Take the lie and rewrite it with truth:

Lie: "I'm disgusting." **Truth:** "I'm a person who deserves respect."

Lie: "It was my fault." **Truth:** "I was a child/young person who was taken advantage of."

Lie: "I'm broken." **Truth:** "I'm healing and growing stronger!"

6. The Daily Counter Each night, write down: One negative thought you caught. Where it came from. One true statement to counter it.

This builds your muscle for recognizing and challenging lies automatically.

Making It Stick: Building New Neural Pathways

Remember neuroplasticity? Here's how to use it to your advantage. Changing thought patterns isn't a one-time thing—it's like going to the gym for your brain. Every repetition builds new neural pathways. Here's how to make the new patterns stronger than the old ones:

Start Small: Pick one lie to focus on this week. Maybe it's "I'm not good enough." Every time you catch it, counter with your truth. You're literally building a new highway in your brain.

Use Reminders: Put sticky notes where you'll see them—your mirror, your notebook, your phone case. Write simple truths: "I am enough" or "Not my fault." Each time you see and read these, you're strengthening new neural pathways.

Create a Truth Playlist: Make a playlist of songs that make you feel strong, worthy, or understood. Music activates multiple parts of your brain at once, making it one of the fastest ways to create new neural pathways.

Practice Self-Compassion: When you catch yourself in old patterns, don't beat yourself up. Say: "There's that old thought again. I'm building new pathways." This self-compassion actually helps your brain change faster than self-criticism.

Track Your Wins: Notice when you successfully challenge a lie. Celebrate it. Your brain releases dopamine when you acknowledge progress, which helps cement the new pathways.

The 5-4-3-2-1 Technique: When negative thoughts spiral, ground yourself: Name 5 things you see, 4 you can touch, 3 you can hear, 2 you can smell, 1 you can taste. This activates different parts of your brain and can interrupt the negative thought loop.

Somatic Exercise for Thought Interruption: When you catch a negative thought, try this: Gently tap your collar bones with your fingertips while taking deep breaths. This bilateral stimulation can help your brain process and release the thought rather than getting stuck in it.

The Science of Change

Here's what's happening in your brain as you do this work:

• **Weakening Old Pathways:** Every time you don't follow the old thought pattern, those neural connections get weaker. It's like a path through the woods that starts to grow over when no one uses it.

• **Building New Pathways:** Every time you choose a different thought, you're laying down new neural connections. At first it's just a thread, but with repetition it becomes a rope, then a bridge.

• **Changing Brain Chemistry:** Practicing self-compassion and challenging negative thoughts actually changes the chemicals your brain produces. Less cortisol (stress), more serotonin and dopamine (well-being).

• **Growing Gray Matter:** Studies show that practices like mindfulness and self-compassion actually increase gray matter in areas of the brain associated with emotional regulation and self-awareness. Gray matter is the brain tissue that contains most of your brain cells and is where information processing happens—think of it as the brain's "working tissue" that handles thinking, decision-making, and emotional responses.

Why This Work Matters

Every time you challenge one of these lies, you're not just changing a thought—you're literally rewiring your brain. You're creating new neural pathways that lead to self-compassion instead of self-hatred. You're taking back control of your own story.

These thoughts might have protected you once by helping you make sense of something senseless. But now they're holding you back from seeing your true worth. You deserve to know the truth about yourself: that you're valuable, that you're worthy of love, that what happened to you doesn't define who you are.

One in three girls and one in six boys experience sexual abuse. Many of them carry these same lying thoughts. You're not alone in this struggle, and you're not alone in learning to fight back.

Moving Forward

The thoughts you're thinking aren't really yours—they're echoes of trauma. But the work you're doing to challenge them? That's all you. That's your strength, your courage, your determination to see yourself clearly.

Some days, the lies will feel louder than the truth. That's okay. Healing isn't linear. Just keep catching those thoughts, checking their source, and countering with compassion. Over time, the truth will get louder and the lies will lose their power.

Remember: your brain's ability to change is lifelong. No matter how long you've believed these lies, no matter how deep those grooves feel, you can create new pathways. Every moment is a chance to choose a different thought, to strengthen a new neural pathway, to become more of who you really are.

You are not your thoughts. You are not what happened to you. You are a person of value, deserving of kindness—especially from yourself. Keep practicing. Keep challenging. Keep choosing truth.

The lies had their time. Now it's time for the truth to win.

Coaching Corner: You Are the Author Now

Those thoughts that feel so true? Someone else wrote them in your story without your permission. But here's the powerful truth: you're the author now. Every time you challenge a lie with truth, you're taking back the pen. Every kind thought toward yourself is a new sentence in your story. Yes, someone else wrote some painful chapters, but they don't get to write your ending. That's your job now, and you're already doing it—one rewritten thought at a time.

10

Triggers and Flashbacks: Managing Overwhelming Moments

Healing isn't about avoiding triggers forever. It's about building a life where they don't control you anymore.

HAVE YOU EVER BEEN going about your day when suddenly—BAM—you're not really there anymore? Maybe a smell, a sound, or even just a feeling catapults you back to the worst moment of your life. Your heart races, your body freezes or wants to run, and you feel like you're right back in that terrible moment, even though you know you're safe now.

Grounding During Flashbacks: When triggered, your body thinks the trauma is happening now. The grounding techniques from Chapter 1—especially feeling your feet on the floor and the 5-4-3-2-1 technique—can help signal safety to your nervous system.

If this happens to you, you're not going crazy. You're experiencing flashbacks or being triggered—totally normal responses to trauma that can make you feel totally out of control. This chapter is about understanding what's happening in these moments and learning tools to bring yourself back to safety, including dealing with the especially tough challenge of nighttime triggers and sleep.

When Your Body Gets Stuck in Survival Mode

Before we dive into triggers and flashbacks, you need to understand what's really happening when these intense reactions occur. Trauma isn't just a bad memory—it's your nervous system getting stuck in survival mode long after the danger has passed. Your body continues to react as if the abuse is still happening, even years later.

This shows up as:

Constant alertness (hypervigilance) - You're always scanning for threats even in safe spaces like your apartment or workplace

Difficulty relaxing or sleeping - Your body won't "turn off" because it thinks it needs to stay ready for danger

Overreacting to small things - Loud noises, unexpected touch, or someone's tone feels like a major threat

Feeling numb or disconnected - Your body shuts down emotions to protect you from feeling too much

People-pleasing - Any tension or conflict feels dangerous, so you avoid it at all costs

Always "waiting for the other shoe to drop" - A constant sense that something bad is about to happen

This isn't a choice you're making. This isn't weakness. This is your brilliant nervous system doing what it learned to do to keep you alive. But what once saved you is now limiting your ability to truly live.

Why Triggers Hit So Hard

When you're stuck in survival mode, your nervous system is already on high alert. So when something reminds your brain of the trauma—a smell, sound, or situation—it doesn't just think "this is similar to what happened before." It screams "THE DANGER IS HAPPENING AGAIN RIGHT NOW!"

That's why triggers feel so intense and why flashbacks feel so real. Your body is responding to a present-moment threat that only exists in your nervous system's memory.

The goal isn't to "get over" trauma or never be triggered again. The goal is to help your body learn that it's safe to come out of survival mode. Every time you use a grounding technique, every time you remind yourself "that was then, this is now," you're teaching your nervous system that the immediate danger is over.

What Are Triggers and Flashbacks?

A trigger is anything that reminds your brain of the trauma—consciously or unconsciously. It could be a smell like cologne or a specific detergent. It might be a sound such as a voice tone, a song, or a door closing. It could be a sight like someone who looks similar, a place, or a color. It might be a sensation like being touched a certain way or feeling trapped. It could be a situation such as being alone with someone or feeling powerless. It might even be a time of day or season.

When you encounter a trigger, your brain doesn't just remember the trauma—it reacts like the trauma is happening again right now. This is because trauma memories get stored differently than regular memories. They're filed in the "immediate danger" section of your brain instead of the "past events" section.

A flashback is when a trigger causes you to re-experience the trauma. Flashbacks can be emotional, where you suddenly feel the terror, shame, or helplessness you felt then. They can be physical, with your body reacting like it did during the trauma with freezing, heart racing, or feeling sick. They might be visual, where you see images or scenes from what happened. Or they can be full flashbacks where you feel like you're completely back in that moment

You might not even realize you're having a flashback. You might just feel "off" or overwhelmed without knowing why.

Nya's Story: When the Past Won't Stay Past

Let me share Nya's story to show you how triggers and flashbacks work—and how to manage them.

Nya was 16 when her manager at the coffee shop started making her uncomfortable. At 24 now, working in marketing, she thought she'd moved on. She never reported what happened—who would have believed her against the popular manager everyone loved? She just quit and found another job.

But certain things would send her into a tailspin. Walking into Star-bucks and smelling that specific coffee blend would make her chest tighten and her breathing shallow. Hearing her boss's voice in team meetings—that same confident, joking tone—would make her zone out completely, missing entire conversations. She'd find herself nod-ding along to meetings she couldn't remember, panic rising as she realized she'd mentally "left" again.

The sound of the espresso machine at work events would transport her back to that cramped break room, feeling trapped and small. Her body would freeze up just like it did at 16, even though she was now a confident adult with her own apartment, car, and career.

Nya started making excuses to avoid work events, turning down pro-motions that required more face-time with leadership. She'd lie awake at night replaying conversations, wondering if she'd missed something important during one of her "episodes."

The hardest part was feeling alone with it. She couldn't explain to her coworkers why she sometimes spaced out in meetings or why she avoided the office coffee machine. Nya thought she should be "over it" by now—it was eight years ago, and she was successful despite it. But her nervous system was still protecting her from a danger that no longer existed.

Learning about triggers helped Nya realize she wasn't weak or crazy. Her brain was just doing its job—keeping her safe from what it per-ceived as ongoing threat.

Why Your Brain Does This

Your brain's number one job is keeping you alive. When you experience trauma, your brain creates a detailed file of everything about that dangerous situation—sights, sounds, smells, feelings—so it can warn you if it ever happens again.

The problem is, your trauma-alert system is super sensitive. It's like a smoke alarm that goes off when you make toast. Your brain thinks it's helping by screaming "DANGER!" but you're actually safe now.

During a flashback, the logical part of your brain (that knows what year it is and that you're safe) goes offline. The survival part takes over, flooding your body with stress chemicals and preparing you to fight, flee, or freeze—just like during the original trauma.

This isn't weakness. It's actually your brain being overprotective. Understanding this can help you be more patient with yourself when it happens.

Recognizing When You're Triggered

Sometimes triggers are obvious—you know exactly what set you off. But often they're sneaky. Here are signs you might be triggered:

Body Signals include heart racing or pounding, sweating or feeling suddenly cold, shaking or trembling, nausea or stomach pain, feeling frozen or unable to move, and muscle tension or pain.

Mind Signals include racing thoughts or mind going blank, feeling disconnected from reality, confusion about where or when you are, overwhelming emotions that don't match the situation, and urges to run, hide, or disappear.

Behavioral Signals include sudden anger or irritability, withdrawing or going silent, overreacting to small things, avoiding certain people, places, or situations, and self-harm urges or behaviors.

Reconnecting After Dissociation: Flashbacks often cause disconnection from your body. Use the gentle body scanning techniques from Chapter 1 to slowly reconnect. If you feel very numb or "outside your body," the body awareness exercises can help you feel grounded again.

Tools for Managing Flashbacks

When you're in a flashback, you need to help your brain realize you're safe in the present. Here are tools that work:

1. The 5-4-3-2-1 Grounding Technique This brings you back to the present by engaging your senses. Name 5 things you can see. Name 4 things you can touch and touch them. Name 3 things you can hear. Name 2 things you can smell. Name 1 thing you can taste.

2. The Time and Place Reminder Say out loud or write down "My name is [your name]," "I am [your age] years old," "I am in [location]," "The date is [today's date]," and "I am safe now."

3. Temperature Shock Use temperature to jolt your nervous system. Hold ice cubes, splash cold water on your face, take a hot shower, or step outside into different air.

4. Movement and Breath Get your body out of freeze mode. Shake your hands and arms vigorously, do jumping jacks, take slow deep breaths with a count of in for 4, hold for 4, out for 6, and walk around while feeling your feet on the ground.

5. Safe Person or Object Have a plan for comfort. Text a friend without needing to explain, just connect. Hold a comfort object like a stuffed animal, smooth stone, or soft fabric. Look at photos that make you feel safe or listen to a specific playlist you've created for these moments.

Somatic Exercise for Flashback Interruption: Try the "Voo" breath from Chapter 6. Take a deep breath and on the exhale, make a low "Voooooo" sound, feeling the vibration in your chest. This activates your vagus nerve and can help shift you out of flashback mode. The vibration is grounding and the sound gives your brain something concrete to focus on.

When Nighttime Is the Hardest

For many survivors, nighttime and sleep are especially challenging. Your defenses are down, the world is quiet, and your brain has time to wander into dangerous territory. If you were hurt at night or in bed, just trying to sleep can feel threatening.

Common nighttime struggles include being unable to fall asleep because you're hypervigilant, having nightmares that feel incredibly real, waking up panicked and disoriented, needing lights on or specific conditions to feel safe, and avoiding sleep altogether.

Creating a Sleep Safety Plan

Before Bed Routine Journal your worries to get them out of your head. Do gentle stretches or breathing exercises. Listen to calming music, meditation apps, or sleep podcasts. Take a warm shower or bath. Say a safety mantra such as "I am safe in my space. That was then, this is now."

Your Sleep Environment Use a nightlight, salt lamp, or soft lighting, there no shame in needing light. Keep comfort items nearby like a weighted blanket, stuffed animal, or soft pillow. Play white noise, nature sounds, or sleep playlists. Make sure your space feels secure with locked doors and familiar surroundings. Keep your phone charged and nearby.

The Nightmare Recovery Plan Turn on a light immediately. Plant your feet on the floor. Hold your comfort object. Drink cold water. Read your safety reminders. Do the 5-4-3-2-1 grounding technique.

Create Safety Reminders: Write these on your phone or on a card by your bed: "I am safe in my space," "That was a dream/memory, not happening now," "I survived the actual thing, I can survive the memory," and "I know what to do to feel better."

Building Your Trigger Management Plan

You can't always avoid triggers, but you can prepare for them:

1. Map Your Triggers Keep a simple log in your phone or journal. Note what happened right before you felt triggered. Record what you noticed in your body. Track what helped you feel better. Look for patterns without judgment—this is just information.

2. Create Coping Strategies For each major trigger, develop responses such as "When I smell [trigger], I remember I'm safe now," "This feeling will pass," and "I can use [specific coping tool]."

3. Build Your Toolkit Assemble things that help including portable grounding objects like fidget toys, smooth stones, or stress balls. Gather scents that calm you such as essential oil roll-ons or favorite lotions. Create playlists that make you feel strong or calm. Keep photos that remind you of safety and joy.

4. Practice When Calm Practice your coping tools when you're not triggered. Your brain needs to know these tools well enough to use them when you're panicked.

Talking to Others (If You Choose To)

You don't have to tell anyone about your trauma to get support with triggers. You can say • "I sometimes have anxiety attacks. If it happens, please give me space." • "Loud noises really affect me. Can we keep the volume reasonable?" • "I need to sit where I can see the door. It helps me feel comfortable." • "Sometimes I zone out during meetings. I'm okay, I just need a minute."

Good friends and colleagues won't need detailed explanations. They'll just want to help you feel comfortable.

The Long-Term Journey

Triggers and flashbacks usually get less intense over time, especially as you practice managing them. Some things that help long-term include regular use of coping strategies, building positive associations (new safe memories in triggering places), physical exercise to discharge trauma energy, creative expression (art, music, writing), and eventually, if you choose, trauma-focused therapy.

Remember: having triggers doesn't mean you're weak or broken. It means you survived something difficult, and your brain is still trying to protect you. Every time you use a coping tool, you're teaching your brain that you're safe now.

You're Stronger Than You Know

Flashbacks and triggers can make you feel powerless, just like you felt during the trauma. But here's the difference: now you have tools. Now you have knowledge. Now you have choices.

You survived the actual trauma. You can survive the memories of it. Each time you ground yourself, each time you remind your brain that you're safe, each time you choose a healthy coping strategy—you're reclaiming your power.

Some days will be harder than others. Some triggers might catch you completely off guard. That's okay. Healing isn't about never being triggered; it's about knowing you can handle it when you are.

You don't have to face this alone. Whether it's a trusted friend, a hotline (RAINN: 1-800-656-HOPE or text RAINN to 741741), or just the knowledge that other survivors understand—support exists when you're ready.

Your triggers don't control you. Your flashbacks don't define you. You're learning to be the author of your own story, one coping skill at a time.

Coaching Corner: Triggers as Teachers

I know triggers feel like enemies, but what if I told you they can become teachers? Every trigger is your body saying, "I remember danger here." Thank your body for trying to protect you, then gently show it the truth: "That was then, this is now. We survived, and we're safe." Over time, triggers lose their power not because you fight them, but because you listen to what they're trying to tell you and respond with compassion. You're not broken for having triggers—you're human, and you're healing.

PART III: BUILDING HEALING PRACTICES

Tools and Techniques for Recovery

11

Building Self-Worth: You Are Enough

Your worth is not determined by what happened to you. It's determined by the simple, profound fact that you exist.

I F YOU'VE EVER LOOKED in the mirror and thought "I'm worthless," or felt like the abuse somehow made you "less than" everyone else, this chapter is especially for you. That feeling—like your value was stolen along with your innocence—is something I carried for years. It's heavy and it hurts, and it feels so real.

But here's what I've learned: your worth was never touched by what happened to you. It's still there, whole and complete, just maybe buried under layers of shame and hurt. This chapter is about excavating that worth, one small dig at a time, and learning to see yourself the way you deserve to be seen—as valuable, important, and absolutely enough.

Understanding Your Worth

Self-worth isn't about what you do, what you achieve, or what happens to you. It's simpler than that: you have worth because you exist.

Period. You were created valuable, and nothing—absolutely nothing—can change that fundamental truth.

I know that might sound like empty words right now. When trauma happens, especially sexual abuse, it can feel like your worth was something that could be taken, used up, or destroyed. The person who hurt you might have acted like you didn't matter. They might have said things that made you feel worthless. The shame that followed might have convinced you that you're "damaged goods."

But here's the truth I wish I'd known sooner: abusers don't have the power to determine your worth. They can hurt your body. They can mess with your mind. They can make you feel worthless. But they cannot actually make you worthless. There's a difference between feeling something and being something.

Why Self-Worth Feels Impossible After Abuse

Sexual abuse attacks your sense of self at the deepest level. Here's why rebuilding worth feels so hard.

The Power Dynamic: Abuse is about power and control. When someone treats you like an object, like your feelings and boundaries don't matter, it's easy to internalize that message. Being treated like you didn't have the right to say no can teach you that you don't matter.

The Shame Factor: Shame tells you that you ARE bad, not just that something bad happened to you. It's like a dark filter over everything, making you see yourself as less than human. That feeling of being tainted, like everyone can somehow see your shame, erodes your sense of worth.

The Secrecy: Keeping abuse secret can make you feel like you're hiding who you really are. You might think, "If people knew the real me, they'd be disgusted." This forced split between your public self and private pain can destroy your sense of inherent value.

The Body Betrayal: If your body responded during abuse (which is just biology, not consent), you might feel like your own body proved you're "bad." This is one of the cruelest lies trauma tells.

The Comparison Trap: Looking at others who seem "normal" or "innocent" can make you feel like you're fundamentally different, like you're marked somehow. But trauma doesn't make you less than—it makes you a survivor.

Sofia's Story: Finding Worth Again

Let me tell you about Sofia, whose journey shows what rebuilding self-worth can look like.

Sofia was 19 when she started dating Ryan, who was 22. He seemed so cool, so charming—the kind of guy who always had a crowd around him at college parties, who could make even the professors laugh with his quick wit. His confidence was magnetic, the way he carried himself through campus like he owned it. Sofia felt chosen, special, when he noticed her among all the other girls who seemed so much more experienced.

But soon he was pressuring her for things she wasn't ready for. His voice would drop to that persuasive tone when they were alone in his dorm room after study sessions, and she'd find herself staring out at the quad while he spoke. "If you really loved me," he'd say, his fingers already reaching, ignoring the way she pulled back. "Everyone else does it." When she tried to say no, he'd get angry—that charming smile disappearing into something cold and hard—or give her the silent treatment until she gave in, desperate to bring back the boy who made her feel special.

Afterward, Sofia felt hollow, like something essential had been scooped out of her chest. Ryan acted like it was no big deal, scrolling through his phone while she sat on his narrow dorm bed feeling like she might dissolve. His casual attitude made her feel worse—was she being dramatic? Was something wrong with her for feeling so awful about what everyone else seemed to think was normal?

By 20, Sofia had internalized a deep belief: "I'm not worth respect. I'm not worth listening to. I'm not enough." She quit the debate team, convincing herself she didn't deserve to be there, that the other students must see right through her to the broken person underneath. She stopped wearing her favorite bright clothes—the yellow sweater that used to make her feel confident, the red dress that brought out her eyes—trying to become invisible, shrinking into oversized hoodies and muted colors. When she looked in the mirror, all she saw was someone who'd "given in," someone weak and worthless.

But then something shifted. Sofia was scrolling through social media one night, curled up in her apartment feeling particularly low, when she saw a post from an account about trauma recovery. The image was simple—just text on a soft background that said: "You are not what happened to you. You are not what they told you. You are not what you tell yourself in your darkest moments. You are worthy simply because you exist."

Sofia stared at those words, reading them over and over until they blurred through her tears. She screenshotted them, saved them to a folder she labeled "maybe true." Something cracked open inside her—not hope exactly, but curiosity. What if the voice in her head was wrong? What if she'd been believing lies?

She started following more accounts about healing, reading stories from other survivors who described feelings she recognized. She found a podcast about trauma and self-worth where the host said, "Would you tell a five-year-old they were worthless because someone hurt them? Then why do you tell yourself that?" Sofia paused the episode and cried—really cried—for the first time in months. She wouldn't tell a child that. So why was she so cruel to herself?

That became Sofia's turning point. She started small—writing down one thing she did well each day in a small notebook she kept on her nightstand. "I helped my study partner understand calculus." "I was patient with my roommate when she was stressed." "I made my mom laugh during our phone call." Tiny things, but they were true, and seeing them written in her own handwriting made them feel more real.

She began standing taller, literally. She'd noticed she was always hunched over, trying to take up less space, shoulders curved inward like she was protecting something precious. So she practiced standing with her shoulders back in front of her bedroom mirror, taking deep breaths, telling herself "I deserve to take up space."

The biggest shift came when Sofia realized that her worth wasn't about being perfect or never making mistakes. It was just about being human.

And humans—all humans—have inherent worth that can't be taken away, even by someone who claims to love you.

How Low Self-Worth Shows Up

After abuse, low self-worth can infiltrate every part of your life.

In How You Treat Yourself: You might engage in negative self-talk that's cruel and constant, neglect basic self-care, punish yourself for normal mistakes, and believe you don't deserve good things.

In Relationships: This shows up as accepting poor treatment because you think it's all you deserve, people-pleasing to earn worth, avoiding relationships because you feel unlovable, and giving too much to "earn" love.

In Daily Life: You might find yourself shrinking—your voice, presence, and opinions—avoiding opportunities because you "don't deserve" them, perfectionism (trying to earn worth through achievement), and self-sabotage when good things happen.

In Your Body: Low self-worth often manifests as avoiding mirrors, hiding under baggy clothes, feeling disconnected from your physical self, and treating your body poorly.

After abuse, many survivors become perfectionists, thinking if they could just be good enough, they'd earn the worth they lost. But worth isn't earned—it just is.

Practical Tools for Building Worth

Physical Self-Compassion: Self-criticism often shows up as body tension, shallow breathing, or numbness. When practicing self-compassion exercises, notice what happens in your body. The body awareness practices from Chapter 1 can help you recognize and shift physical patterns of self-judgment.

You don't need to believe you're worthy yet. You just need to act like someone who has worth, and slowly, your brain will catch up. Here are tools that actually work:

1. The Daily Worth Evidence List: Each day, write three pieces of evidence that you have worth—kind things you did (even tiny ones), challenges you faced (getting out of bed counts), and positive impacts you had (making someone smile). Start small. "I fed my pet" counts. "I didn't give up" counts.

2. The Mirror Challenge: This is hard but powerful. Look yourself in the eyes in a mirror and say out loud "I have worth," "I deserve respect," and "I am enough." It will feel fake at first. Do it anyway. Your brain needs to hear these words in your own voice.

3. The Friend Test: When your inner critic attacks, ask: "Would I say this to my best friend?" If not, you don't deserve to hear it either. Practice being as kind to yourself as you'd be to someone you care about.

4. Physical Worth-Building: Your body language affects your feelings. Practice standing tall with shoulders back, taking up space when you sit, speaking at a normal volume (not shrinking your voice), and making eye contact. Your body teaches your brain: "I deserve to exist fully."

5. Worth Affirmations That Don't Feel Cheesy: Instead of "I'm amazing!" try realistic affirmations like "I'm learning to value myself," "My worth isn't determined by my past," "I'm allowed to take up space," and "I deserve basic human respect."

6. The Worth Jar: Get a jar or box. Every time you do something kind, brave, or just human, write it on a paper and add it to the jar. When you feel worthless, read the words you wrote. Physical evidence helps combat lies.

7. Boundary Practice: Start with tiny boundaries like saying "no thanks" to food you don't want, asking for a few minutes before responding to texts, and choosing what movie to watch. Each boundary tells your brain: "My preferences matter. I matter."

Somatic Exercise for Building Worth: Stand with your feet hip-width apart. Place both hands over your heart. Take a deep breath and as you exhale, gently press your hands into your chest while saying internally "I matter." Feel the warmth and pressure of your own hands. This physical self-compassion helps your nervous system integrate the message of worth.

Reframing Your Story

One powerful way to build worth is to reframe how you see your story:

Instead of "I let it happen," try "I survived something terrible." Instead of "I'm damaged," try "I'm healing from injury." Instead of "I'm weak," try "I'm strong enough to keep going." Instead of "I'm worthless," try "My worth was hidden, not destroyed."

You're not rewriting history or pretending everything's fine. You're choosing to see your story through a lens of compassion rather than shame.

Dealing with Worth Attacks

Some days, no matter how much work you've done, those "I'm worthless" feelings will hit hard. Here's an emergency plan: Acknowledge it by saying "I'm having a worth attack right now." Remember it's temporary by telling yourself "This feeling will pass." Use your evidence by reading your worth lists or jar. Do one kind thing for yourself, no matter how small. Reach out by texting a friend, even just to say "hey." Move your body since worth attacks often freeze us and gentle movement helps.

The Long Game of Worth

Building self-worth after abuse isn't a quick fix. It's like physical therapy after an injury—slow, sometimes painful, but absolutely possible. Here's what to expect:

It's not linear: Some days you'll feel worthy, others you won't. That's normal, not failure.

Old patterns die hard: You might catch yourself accepting poor treatment or shrinking yourself. Noticing is the first step to changing.

Worth attracts worth: As you value yourself more, you'll naturally attract people who value you too. You'll also notice toxic people faster.

It compounds: Each small act of self-worth builds on the last. It gets easier over time.

Why This Matters So Much

Your worth isn't just some feel-good concept. It affects everything: how you let others treat you, what opportunities you pursue, how you care for your body and mind, whether you seek help when needed, and your entire future.

When you finally start believing you have worth, everything changes. You stop accepting crumbs in relationships. You pursue goals you thought were "too good" for you. You learn to say no without guilt. You discover that you deserve to heal, not just survive.

A Personal Note

I want to tell you something I wish someone had told me when I was drowning in worthlessness: You are not what happened to you. You are not the lies trauma told you. You are not too damaged, too dirty, or too broken for good things.

You are a human being who survived something no one should have to survive. That makes you incredibly strong, not worthless. Every day you keep going, every time you choose to try building your worth instead of giving up—that's heroic.

Your worth was there when you were born. It was there during the worst moments. It's there right now as you read this. And it will be there tomorrow and every day after. Nothing and no one can take it away—they can only convince you to stop seeing it.

But you're starting to see it again, aren't you? Even if it's just a glimmer. That's enough to start. That glimmer will grow into a flame if you keep tending it with small acts of self-worth.

You are enough. You've always been enough. And one day, you'll not only know that in your mind—you'll feel it in your bones.

Coaching Corner: The Worth You Were Born With

Picture a newborn baby. Would you ever say that baby has to earn worth? Would you say they need to achieve something to deserve love? Of course not. That baby has infinite worth simply by existing. Here's the secret: that's still true about you. The part of you that has worth is the same part that had worth as a baby—your existence itself. Yes, life has been hard. Yes, people have treated you badly. But that original worth? It's still there, untouched, waiting for you to remember it. You don't need to earn it. You just need to uncover it.

12

Reclaiming Your Identity After Trauma

You are not what happened to you. You are who you choose to become.

S O WE'VE TALKED ABOUT shame—how it lies to you, makes you feel like you're fundamentally flawed or broken. But here's the thing: if shame isn't who you are (and it's not), then who are you really?

That's what this chapter is about. Because when trauma happens—especially when you're young—it doesn't just hurt you. It confuses you about who you are. Instead of growing up confident in your identity, you grow up wondering if you're even worth knowing.

Maybe you've spent years letting other people define you. Maybe you've believed every cruel thing your brain tells you about yourself. Maybe you look in the mirror and honestly don't know who's looking back.

If you've never told anyone about your abuse, or if you tried and weren't believed, this identity confusion runs even deeper. You might not even connect your struggles with relationships, your self-doubt, or that constant feeling of being "different" to what happened to you.

But here's what I know: trauma may be part of your story, but it is not your identity. You are so much more than what someone did to you.

Why Your Identity Matters So Much

When you don't know who you are, everyone else gets to decide for you. Every rejection feels like proof you're worthless. Every mistake confirms you're a failure. Every cruel word sticks because you don't have a strong sense of self to push back against it.

That's exhausting. And it's exactly what trauma wants—to keep you small, confused, unsure of your own worth.

But identity isn't about what people say about you. It's not even about what you've done or what's been done to you. It's about discovering (or rediscovering) who you really are underneath all the pain and confusion.

The exercises in this chapter aren't about "fixing" yourself—you were never broken. They're about remembering and reclaiming what was always yours.

Exercise 1: The Mirror Letter

This one might feel weird at first, but stick with me.

What You'll Do: Sit somewhere quiet where you won't be interrupted. Imagine standing in front of a mirror, looking into the eyes of someone who's survived incredible pain—you. Now write a letter to that person in the mirror. Talk to yourself like you would talk to your best friend who's hurting.

Start like this: *"Dear [Your name], I see you. I know you've been through things that no one should have to go through. Things that tried to break you. And yet here you are, still standing, still fighting, still trying..."*

Keep writing. Tell yourself what you see when you look at this survivor in the mirror, what you admire about how they've made it this far, what they need to hear today, and what hopes you have for their future.

Why This Works: We're often way meaner to ourselves than we'd ever be to someone else. This exercise helps you practice self-compassion by creating a little distance—you're writing TO yourself, not AS yourself. It bypasses that harsh inner critic.

Tips: Include specific things you love about yourself (even tiny things count). Acknowledge the pain without letting it be the whole story. End with something hopeful, even if it's small. If you cry while writing this, that's okay. Tears can be healing too.

Exercise 2: Circles of Identity

Trauma makes everything feel jumbled together—like your whole identity is just "person who was hurt." This exercise helps you see that you're actually made up of many layers, and trauma only touched some of them.

What You'll Do: Draw three circles inside each other (like a target). Each circle represents a different part of who you are:

Innermost Circle - Your Core Self This is the deepest, truest part of you. The stuff that can't be taken away. Write words that describe who you are at your core: creative, curious, loyal, resilient, kind, fighter, dreamer, deep thinker.

Middle Circle - Your Connections & Values This is how you relate to the world—your roles, passions, the things you care about: friend, big sister or brother, music lover, animal person, gamer, writer, advocate, introvert or extrovert, nature lover.

Outer Circle - Your Experiences & Labels This is stuff that's happened to you or labels you've carried: survivor, student, anxious, trauma survivor, perfectionist, people pleaser, depressed.

Now Look at Your Drawing: Notice how trauma is just one thing in the outer circle? It's something you experienced, not who you are at your core. Your innermost circle—your true self—remains untouched. Trauma couldn't reach that deep.

Exercise 3: The "I Am / I Am Not" List

Trauma plants lies in your head about who you are. This exercise helps you fight back with truth.

What You'll Do: Make two columns on a page. In the left column, write "I AM" statements—truths about who you really are. In the right column, write "I AM NOT" statements—lies that trauma wants you to believe.

I AM: I am worthy of love and respect. I am healing, even when it doesn't feel like it. I am stronger than I know. I am allowed to take up space. I am learning to trust again. I am creative and capable. I am allowed to say no. I am becoming who I was meant to be. I am enough, exactly as I am. I am brave for still being here.

I AM NOT: I am not what happened to me. I am not broken or damaged goods. I am not responsible for someone else's choices. I am not too much or too little. I am not alone, even when I feel lonely. I am not defined by my worst moments. I am not stuck forever. I am not worthless. I am not a burden. I am not done growing.

Make It Yours: Add to this list whenever you need to. When shame whispers a lie, write its opposite truth. When someone's words sting, counter them with who you really are. Keep this list somewhere you can see it—on your phone, by your mirror, wherever you need the reminder.

The Power of Your Name: Discovering Hidden Identity

One of the most powerful exercises I do with clients might sound simple at first, but it often brings people to tears. I ask them to research what their name means—first, middle, and last—and create what I call their "Signature Statement" or "Personal Creed."

I'll never forget Sarah (not her real name), who came to me convinced she was worthless. Years of abuse had taught her that her identity was "victim," "damaged," "unwanted." She could barely make eye contact during our first sessions.

When I asked her to look up her names, she rolled her eyes. "What's the point? A name is just what people call you."

But she did it anyway. That next week, she came back with trembling hands and tears in her eyes.

"My first name means 'princess,'" she whispered. "My middle name means 'pure lily.' And my last name means 'fortress on the hill.'"

We sat with that for a moment. This woman who felt dirty, worthless, and defenseless discovered she was named "Pure Princess, Fortress on the Hill."

Together, we crafted her Signature Statement: "Royal in worth, pure in essence, standing strong on solid ground."

She wrote it on a card and carried it everywhere. When shame attacked, she'd pull out that card and whisper her true identity. Not the identity trauma gave her, but the one she'd carried all along, hidden in the very name she'd been called since birth.

Creating Your Own Signature Statement

Your name holds more power than you might realize. Many believe names carry destiny, that they're chosen with divine purpose. Whether you see it that way or not, discovering what your name means can unlock a new way of seeing yourself.

Creating Your Own Signature Statement

Your name holds more power than you might realize. Many believe names carry destiny, that they're chosen with divine purpose. Whether you see it that way or not, discovering what your name means can unlock a new way of seeing yourself. Here are the steps to create your own and some examples to get you started.

Step 1: Research Your Names Look up each of your names (first, middle, last) on name meaning websites like Behind the Name, Nameberry, or in name books. Write down all the meanings—sometimes names have multiple origins or interpretations. Don't worry if some meanings seem ordinary; focus on what resonates.

Step 2: Identify Your Power Words From all the meanings, circle the words that feel significant to you. Look for qualities like:

Strength words (warrior, fortress, defender)

Beauty words (light, grace, beloved)

Character words (noble, wise, faithful)

Nature words (flower, mountain, flowing water)

Step 3: Create Your Statement Pattern Use one of these formats:

"I am [quality] in [area], [quality] in [area], [action/state]"

"[Quality descriptor], [character trait], [position of strength]"

"Born to be [calling], gifted with [attribute], standing as [identity]"

Examples

Esperanza (hope - Spanish), Marie (wished for child - Hebrew), Garcia (bear/brave - Spanish) = "Born of hope, treasured and wanted, courageously strong .

David (beloved), Hope (expectation), Rivers (flowing water) = "Deeply loved, living with hope, flowing forward with purpose"

Peyton (fighting man's estate), Colby (dark village), Ortiz (son of fortune) = "Warrior by nature, emerging from shadows, blessed with favor"

Step 4: Make It Personal Adjust the wording until it feels like YOU. Your statement should make you stand a little taller when you say it.

Signature Statements examples from my family:

Kyra Lauren Mathley: *Queen in spirit, wise in purpose, legacy in motion.*

Hannah Shae Mathley: *Rooted in grace. Elevated with purpose. Empowered as a cherished legacy.*

Olivia Grace Mathley: *Grace in every step, peace in every season, fruitfulness in every field.*

What If You Don't Like Your Name?

Sometimes trauma is connected to our names—maybe your abuser gave you a nickname, or your name reminds you of pain. That's okay. You can focus on just one name that feels safe, choose the most empowering meaning if multiple exist, create a chosen name that represents your healing, or add a meaningful word that represents your journey.

One client whose name reminded her of her abuser chose to focus on her middle name and added the word "Phoenix" to represent her rising. Her statement became: "Hope rising from ashes, transformed by fire, soaring in freedom."

This isn't about positive thinking or pretending. It's about discovering that maybe, just maybe, your true identity has been with you all along.

Maybe before you were ever hurt, before anyone tried to define you, you were already named with purpose.

Whether you believe your name was chosen with intention or you see it as beautiful coincidence, the meaning you discover can become an anchor. When trauma tries to rename you "worthless," you can respond with your true name. When shame whispers "damaged," you can declare your Signature Statement.

Finding Your True Identity in God's Eyes

While this book focuses on practical healing tools that work regardless of your faith background, many survivors find deep healing in understanding who God says they are—truths that no abuse can ever change.

If you're interested in exploring your identity from a faith perspective, I've included a special supplement at the back of this book called "Who God Says You Are: Unchangeable Truths About Your Identity." These biblical truths have brought profound healing to many survivors, reminding them that their worth and identity were established by their Creator long before anyone tried to harm them. You don't need to embrace faith to heal—the tools in this book stand on their own. But if faith is part of your journey, these truths about your God-given identity might provide additional comfort and strength.

Why This Identity Work Matters

Here's the truth: you might not fully believe these exercises yet. You might write "I am worthy" while everything in you screams that you're not. That's okay. You don't have to feel it to start claiming it.

Think of it like planting seeds. Every time you write or speak these truths about yourself, you're planting something new. It might not sprout immediately. But with time and repetition, these truths will start to take root.

Because the real you—the one who existed before trauma, who exists beyond trauma—is still in there. Strong. Beautiful. Creative. Worthy. Whole. Just waiting to be remembered and reclaimed.

Your Story, Your Authorship

Trauma tried to rewrite your story, to make you forget who you were before it happened. But you get to be the author now. You get to decide what defines you.

And I promise you this: you are so much more than what happened to you. You always have been. You always will be.

You are not what happened to you. You are not what they called you. You are the person your name declares you to be—and that person is worthy, valuable, and designed for purpose.

Keep going. Keep remembering. Keep reclaiming what's yours.

Coaching Corner: The Page as Witness

When no one else saw what happened to you, when no one else validated your pain, the page becomes your witness. It doesn't judge, doesn't minimize, doesn't tell you to "get over it." It simply receives whatever you need to pour out. Every word you write is you saying, "This happened. This mattered. I matter." The page holds space for all the parts of your story—the ugly parts, the painful parts, the parts you can barely think about. And in that holding, something shifts. You're no longer alone with it. The page has seen, and somehow, that changes everything.

13

Healing Through Mindfulness and Meditation

The present moment is the only place where trauma doesn't
exist. Learning to find it is learning to find freedom.

I F YOU'VE EVER FELT like your mind is a hamster wheel of painful memories, or your body is constantly braced for danger even when you're safe, you're not alone. After trauma, it can feel like you're never really "here"—you're either stuck in the past or terrified of the future. I spent years feeling that way after my own abuse, like my mind and body were enemies I couldn't escape.

But here's something that changed everything for me: learning that I could find moments of peace right in the middle of the storm. Mindfulness and meditation aren't about emptying your mind or pretending everything's fine. They're about learning to be present with yourself, even when it's hard. This chapter will show you simple, private ways to find calm in your own mind and body, one breath at a time.

What Mindfulness and Meditation Really Mean

Let's clear something up, mindfulness isn't some mystical thing that requires sitting cross-legged on a mountain. It's simply noticing what's happening right now—in your thoughts, feelings, and body—without judging it as good or bad. It's like being a gentle observer of your own experience.

Meditation is just a formal way of practicing mindfulness. It might mean focusing on your breath, body sensations, or even sounds around you. The goal isn't to stop thinking (impossible) or to feel blissful (unrealistic). It's to give your traumatized nervous system a break from constant alert mode.

Many survivors instinctively find their own forms of mindfulness without realizing it—focusing on breathing when memories get too intense, or staring at a candle flame when sleep won't come. Those moments of focus are your brain's way of trying to find safety. Now we know there's science behind why it helps.

Why Your Traumatized Brain Needs This

Sexual abuse hijacks your nervous system. It leaves you in a constant state of threat detection, even when you're objectively safe. Your amygdala (the brain's alarm system) is like a smoke detector that goes off every time someone makes toast. Exhausting, right?

Mindfulness and meditation work by calming your overactive alarm system, teaching your body it's safe to relax, creating space between you and your thoughts, building your ability to stay present instead of dissociating, and giving you tools that are always available, no matter where you are.

Research shows that regular mindfulness practice actually changes your brain structure, strengthening the parts that help you regulate emotions and weakening the parts that keep you in panic mode. Since brains continue developing until about age 25, this is especially powerful for younger people—you're literally rewiring your brain for calm instead of chaos.

Riley's Story: Finding Quiet in the Storm

Let me tell you about Riley to show how this works in real life.

Riley was 12 when a family friend started making comments that they really didn't understand and touching them during visits. Cal had a way of making everything seem normal and harmless. During family barbecues when the adults were distracted, he'd ask Riley to help him get something from his car or the garage. "Riley's such a good helper," he'd announce to the group, making it seem like a simple favor. Once alone, his touches became inappropriate, but he'd quickly follow with "You know I didn't mean anything by that, right? We're just playing around."

Riley froze every time, their mind spinning with confusion. If this was wrong, why did Cal act so casual about it? If it was normal, why did it feel so horrible? Cal's constant reassurances that "this is what friends do" and "you're so mature for your age" left Riley questioning their own instincts. They wanted to tell someone but couldn't find words for something Cal insisted was perfectly ordinary. Riley worried that adults would think they were overreacting, or worse, that they'd somehow invited this attention by being too friendly or helpful.

By 22, Riley's body was constantly on high alert. Their brain had learned that trusted people could become dangerous without warning, that normal social situations could turn threatening in an instant. Office environments felt like danger zones—too many people who might get too close, too many opportunities for someone to corner them in a hallway or empty conference room. Riley couldn't focus during meetings because their mind was always calculating escape routes and scanning for potential threats. They sat near doors, avoided being alone with colleagues, and felt exhausted from the constant vigilance.

One day, Riley's workplace offered a stress management workshop that included a simple breathing exercise. Riley thought it was pointless at first—how could breathing fix a nervous system that had learned the world was fundamentally unsafe? But something about the rhythm made the constant buzz of anxiety quiet down for just a moment, like someone had turned down the volume on the chaos in their head.

Curious despite their skepticism, they tried it again alone that night in their apartment. At first, sitting still felt impossible. Riley's mind raced with thoughts like "This won't work for someone like me" and "What if I let my guard down and something happens?" But they kept trying, just for 2-3 minutes at a time, reasoning that they could stop immediately if they felt unsafe.

Slowly, they noticed that during those minutes of focused breathing, their hypervigilant mind could rest. They weren't "cured"—the constant scanning was still there, the startled responses still happened—but they'd found a way to give their overtaxed nervous system brief moments of relief. Riley started using mindfulness throughout the day, focusing on their breath when panic started to rise, doing quick grounding exercises when memories intruded. It became their secret tool for managing the hypervigilance that Dave's grooming had embedded in their nervous system, a way to find moments of calm despite their brain's insistence that danger was always near.

Simple Mindfulness Practices for Trauma Survivors

You don't need any special equipment, apps, or training. Here are practices specifically helpful for trauma survivors:

1. The Trauma-Informed Breath

Unlike traditional deep breathing, this is gentler. Start by simply noticing your natural breath without changing it. When you're ready, try counting: In for 4, hold for 4, out for 4. If holding your breath feels triggering, try this instead: In for 4, out for 6. Place a hand on your chest or belly to feel the movement. Do this for just 1-2 minutes to start.

2. The Body Scan (Trauma-Adapted)

Traditional body scans can be triggering when you come to body areas that were violated.so try this modified version. Start with neutral body parts (elbows, knees, ears). Just notice sensations without trying to relax. Skip any body parts that feel unsafe. Keep your eyes open if needed. Stop anytime—you're in control.

3. The 5-4-3-2-1 Present Moment

This grounds you in the here and now. Name 5 things you can see, 4 things you can physically feel (chair, air temperature, etc.), 3 things you can hear, 2 things you can smell, and 1 thing you can taste. This interrupts flashbacks and dissociation.

4. Movement Meditation

If sitting still feels unsafe, try walking slowly while feeling each step on the ground, stretching gently while noticing the sensations in your muscles, dancing to one song while focusing on how your body moves, or doing simple yoga poses while breathing with each movement.

5. The Safe Place Visualization

Create a mental refuge. Picture a place where you feel completely safe. Add details: colors, sounds, smells, temperature. "Visit" this place for a few minutes daily. Use it when you feel overwhelmed. Remember: this place is always available to you.

6. Mindful Daily Activities

Turn routine tasks into mindfulness practices. Brush your teeth noticing every sensation—the bristles, the taste, the movement. Eat one bite of food really slowly, tasting every flavor. Feel the water temperature and pressure during your shower. Notice the sensation of petting an animal, the texture of their fur. These build mindfulness without formal meditation.

Somatic Mindfulness Exercise - Hand Awareness: This is especially good for grounding. Hold your hands in front of you and very slowly open and close them. Notice every sensation—the stretch of your skin, the movement of your joints, the air between your fingers. Do this for 30 seconds. This simple practice brings you fully into your body and the present moment, interrupting trauma loops.

Working with Resistance and Triggers

Sometimes mindfulness can feel scary for trauma survivors. Here's why and what to do:

"I can't stop thinking about the trauma": That's normal. Don't try to stop thoughts. Just notice them like clouds passing by. You can say, "There's that memory again" and gently return to your breath.

"Being still makes me panic": Start with movement-based practices or keep your eyes open. You're not trapped—you can stop anytime.

"I feel nothing/numb": Numbness is a sensation too. Just notice it without judgment. Feeling will return when your nervous system feels safer.

"This is making things worse": Sometimes things feel more intense before they feel better. But if it's truly distressing, stop and try a different practice. You're in charge.

Your Mindfulness Toolkit

Create a personalized plan:

Morning: 2 minutes of breathing before getting out of bed
Midday: One mindful activity (eating, walking or what makes sense in your routine)
Evening: 5-minute body scan or visualization
Emergency: 5-4-3-2-1 grounding when triggered

Start small. Even 30 seconds counts. Consistency matters more than duration.

Orienting Exercise for Safety: When you feel disconnected or unsafe, try this: Slowly look around the room. Name what you see, but add "and I am safe." For example: "I see a blue wall, and I am safe. I see my bedroom door, and I am safe." This combines mindfulness with safety affirmations, helping your nervous system calm down.

Advanced Practices (When You're Ready)

Once basic mindfulness feels comfortable, you might try:

• Loving-kindness meditation (sending good wishes to yourself)
• Apps like Headspace or Calm for guided practices
• Trauma-informed yoga classes
• Progressive muscle relaxation
• Breathwork techniques

Remember: these are tools, not rules. Use what helps, leave what doesn't.

Why This Matters So Much

Every moment you spend in mindfulness, you're teaching your nervous system it's safe to relax, building resilience against triggers, creating space between you and trauma responses, developing a tool that's always available, and literally rewiring your brain for calm.

Mindfulness is like learning to swim when you're drowning in trauma symptoms. At first, you might barely keep your head above water for a few seconds. But those seconds add up. Over time, you learn to float, then swim, then maybe even enjoy the water.

To You, Right Now

I know sitting with yourself can feel terrifying when you're carrying trauma. Your mind might feel like an unsafe place. Your body might feel like enemy territory. But you deserve moments of peace. You deserve to feel safe in your own skin.

Start tiny. One breath. One moment of noticing. You don't have to be good at this. You don't have to feel peaceful. You just have to try, gently and with infinite patience for yourself.

Your trauma taught your nervous system to be hypervigilant. Now you're teaching it something new: that it's safe to rest. That you're okay right now. That this moment, right here, is survivable.

You've already survived the worst. Now it's time to learn to thrive, one mindful moment at a time.

> **Coaching Corner: The Power of Now**
> Trauma lives in the past. Anxiety lives in the future. But you? You live right here, right now, in this moment. And in this exact moment, reading these words, you are safe. Your breath is moving in and out. Your heart is beating. You are alive and you are here. That's mindfulness—not some perfect state of zen, but simply remembering that this moment is the only one that's real. The past already happened. The future isn't here yet. But this breath? This heartbeat? This is yours, and trauma can't touch it.

14

Writing to Heal: Journaling and Expressive Writing

*The page holds what you cannot. It witnesses what no one else
has seen. It gives voice to the silenced parts of you.*

I F YOU'VE EVER FELT like you're choking on words you can't say, like there's a scream trapped in your chest with nowhere to go, I get it. After abuse, many of us feel silenced twice—first by what happened, then by the secret we have to keep. But there's something that can save you: writing. Not perfect writing, not writing for anyone else to read. Just raw, messy, honest writing for you.

I've learned that putting words on paper can be one of the most powerful healing tools we have. It's free, it's private, and it's always available. This chapter will show you how to use writing to process your pain, reclaim your voice, and slowly make sense of what feels senseless.

Why Writing Works When Nothing Else Does

There's something almost magical about transferring pain from your body to paper. Here's what's actually happening:

Your Brain on Writing: Writing organizes chaotic trauma memories, engages both emotional and logical parts of your brain, helps you process experiences your nervous system couldn't handle in the moment, creates distance between you and your pain, and literally changes how memories are stored.

The Power of Privacy: No one needs to read what you write. You can be completely honest without fear. You can destroy it afterward if you want. You control every aspect. There's no "wrong" way to do it.

When survivors first start writing about their abuse, they often can barely form sentences. Just fragments. Single words. Scribbles of rage. But even that helps. It's like opening a pressure valve—suddenly you can breathe a little easier.

Diego's Story: When Words Find a Way Out

Diego sits at his kitchen table at 6:42 AM, laptop open, cursor blinking in the empty document. The coffee has gone cold in his favorite mug—the one with the chip on the handle that his thumb finds automatically. Outside, garbage trucks rumble past his apartment window, their hydraulic whines mixing with the sound of his upstairs neighbor's shower running.

This is his fourth attempt at writing this morning. The first three documents are buried in his trash folder, deleted in frustration after he'd stare at the screen for twenty minutes without typing a single word. But today feels different. Today, the silence in his head doesn't feel as heavy.

It's been eight months since he started therapy with Dr. Chen, eight months since he first said the words "sexual abuse" out loud in her small office that smells like lavender and has too many plants. Eight months since he stopped pretending the rage that lived in his chest was just "stress from work" or "growing up in a tough neighborhood."

Diego's fingers hover over the keyboard. He's not trying to write the Great American Novel. He's not even trying to write something good. Dr. Chen gave him permission to write badly, to let the words come out messy and broken if that's how they want to emerge. He types: "I was five." The words sit there on the screen, black letters against white background, stark and simple. He stares at them, waiting for the usual flood of panic, the urge to delete and close the laptop and pretend he never tried. But his breathing stays steady. His shoulders don't hunch up toward his ears the way they used to. He keeps typing:

"I was five and he was seventeen and I didn't have words for what he did to me in that basement that smelled like fabric softener and something else I couldn't name. I just knew it felt wrong and scary and I couldn't tell anyone because he said it was our secret and secrets were supposed to be special." Diego pauses, takes a sip of cold coffee, grimaces at the bitter taste.

The words are coming easier now, like a dam with a small crack that's finally giving way. "I'm twenty-six now and I'm tired of carrying this alone. I'm tired of the anger that comes out of nowhere when someone stands too close to me on the subway. I'm tired of feeling like I'm different from everyone else, like I have this invisible mark that keeps me separate from normal life."

He writes about the rage that used to consume him, how he'd punch walls until his knuckles bled, how he'd start fights with strangers just to have somewhere to put all that fire. He writes about the shame that followed, the voice in his head that sounded like his own but spoke words that weren't his: "You let it happen. You didn't fight back. What kind of man are you?"

The clock on his laptop says 7:23 AM. Diego has been writing for forty-one minutes, and the document is three pages long. Three pages of truth he's never spoken aloud, not even to Dr. Chen. Not yet. He saves the document—not to share, not to publish, but to keep. Evidence that he survived, that he can name what happened, that the seventeen-year-old in that basement doesn't get to write the end of Diego's story. Tomorrow morning, he'll sit at this same table with another cup of coffee. Maybe he'll write more. Maybe he'll just read what he wrote today and remember that some silences are meant to be broken, some secrets need to be shared, one word at a time.

The Science of Writing Through Trauma

Research shows that expressive writing about trauma reduces intrusive thoughts and nightmares, decreases anxiety and depression, improves immune function (trauma is stored in the body), helps create a coherent narrative from fragmented memories, and increases self-compassion and emotional regulation.

You don't need to understand the science to benefit. You just need a pen and paper (or a phone or computer) and the courage to start.

The Healing Power of Tears: Why Crying is Medicine

Many trauma survivors have learned that crying is "weak," "manipulative," or "dangerous." You might have been told to "stop crying" or that tears made your abuser angry. Perhaps you learned that crying brought unwanted attention, punishment, or made the abuse worse. Maybe you were raised in a family or culture that saw tears as shameful, especially if you're male.

But here's what science tells us: crying is one of your body's most sophisticated healing mechanisms. When you cry, you're not being weak—you're being wise. Your body is doing exactly what it needs to do to heal.

What Happens in Your Body When You Cry

Stress Hormone Release: Your tears aren't just salt water. Emotional tears—the kind that come from pain, grief, or overwhelming feelings—contain actual stress hormones. When you cry, you're literally washing cortisol, adrenaline, and other stress chemicals out of your body through your tear ducts. Think of it like this: trauma floods your system with stress hormones. Your body stores what it can't process. Crying gives these stored chemicals a way out. Each tear carries a little bit of that stored stress away from you.

Natural Pain Relief: When you cry, your brain releases endorphins—your body's natural painkillers. These are the same chemicals released during exercise or laughter. They don't just help with physical pain; they ease emotional pain too. This is why you often feel calmer or even slightly better after a good cry, even when your situation hasn't changed.

Nervous System Reset: Crying activates your parasympathetic nervous system—the part that helps you "rest and digest." When you're stuck in fight-or-flight mode from trauma, crying can be like hitting a reset button. It signals to your nervous system that the immediate danger has passed and it's safe to begin healing.

Emotional Completion: Trauma often happens so fast that your nervous system doesn't get to complete its natural responses. You might have wanted to scream, run, or fight back, but couldn't. Crying can help complete these interrupted responses, allowing your nervous system to finish what it started during the traumatic event.

Why Trauma Survivors Often Can't Cry

If you rarely cry or feel like you "can't" cry, you're not broken. Trauma affects our ability to cry in several ways. When you're constantly scanning for danger, your body suppresses "vulnerable" responses like crying. Your nervous system thinks, "We don't have time for tears—we need to stay alert." If crying brought negative consequences—more abuse, punishment, or being called names—your body learned to shut down the crying response to keep you safe. Some trauma survivors feel disconnected from all emotions, including the ones that trigger tears. This protective numbing can make crying feel impossible. If you're always "on guard," the relaxation required for crying might feel too vulnerable or dangerous. You might fear that if you start crying, you'll never stop, or that crying means you're "losing control."

Different Types of Healing Tears

Not all tears are the same, and they all serve different healing purposes.

Grief Tears come when you're mourning losses—your innocence, your childhood, relationships damaged by trauma, or the person you might have been without trauma. These tears honor what you've lost and help you process the reality of that loss.

Rage Tears sometimes bring anger and tears together. These aren't weak tears—they're powerful tears. They carry the energy of righteous anger about what was done to you. Let them come.

Relief Tears might surprise you. They come when you finally feel safe, when someone believes you, or when you realize you're not alone. Relief tears release the tension you've been holding for so long.

Fear Tears can come with terror. These help discharge the intense energy of fear and can actually help calm your nervous system after overwhelming experiences.

Healing Tears sometimes come during therapy, meditation, or quiet moments for no clear reason. These are your nervous system releasing old, stored emotions. Trust them.

When Crying Feels Dangerous

If the idea of crying terrifies you, start small and stay safe. Choose a private space where you won't be interrupted. Have tissues, water, and comfort items nearby. Consider having a trusted person you can call if needed. Remember you can stop anytime. You don't have to cry "pretty" or quietly. Set a timer if you're worried about crying "too long." You can cry about one specific thing and save other feelings for later. It's okay to cry angry, scared, or confused tears.

If tears won't come, try watching a sad movie or listening to emotional music, looking at old photos that bring up feelings, writing about your pain first (sometimes tears follow words), or trying the body awareness exercises from Chapter 1 to reconnect with feelings.

Supporting Your Tears

During crying, breathe deeply when you can, place your hand on your heart, say kind things to yourself like "It's okay to feel this," "I'm safe now," or "These tears are healing," and let your body move if it wants to—rocking, curling up, or reaching for comfort.

After crying, drink water (crying is dehydrating), rest if you feel tired (emotional release takes energy), be gentle with yourself for the rest of the day, and notice any sense of relief, lightness, or peace that might follow.

Tears as Medicine

Your tears know things your mind doesn't. They carry wisdom about what you need to release, what you're grieving, and what you're healing. When you cry, you're not being "too sensitive"—you're being human. You're not losing control—you're gaining it back. You're not weak—you're incredibly brave. You're not broken—you're healing.

Every tear you allow yourself to shed is an act of self-compassion. It's your body doing what it knows how to do to help you heal. In a world that often tells trauma survivors to "be strong" and "move on," choosing to honor your tears is revolutionary.

Your tears have been waiting for you to feel safe enough to let them flow. They carry messages from your deepest self, and they know exactly how to help you heal. Trust them. Trust yourself. And know that every tear is washing away a little more of what was never yours to carry in the first place.

Your Writing Toolkit: Different Ways to Heal

1. The Feeling Dump: Set a timer for 5–10 minutes and write whatever you're feeling. Don't stop, don't edit, don't judge. If you run out of words, write "I don't know what to write" until more words come. This clears emotional congestion.

2. The Unsent Letter Series: Write letters you'll never send—to the person who hurt you, to yourself at the age it happened, to the people who didn't protect you, to your future healed self, or to other survivors. Say everything you wish you could say. Be angry. Be sad. Be real.

3. The Story Rewrite: Write about your trauma in third person, like it happened to a character in a book. This creates helpful distance. You can even give the character the ending you wish you'd had—fighting back, getting help, being believed.

4. The Daily Check-In: Each day, write one feeling you experienced, one thought that bothered you, one small good thing (even tiny counts), and one thing you're grateful you survived. This builds awareness and self-compassion over time.

5. The Body Scan Journal: Write what you notice in your body—where you hold tension, what feels numb, what feels painful, and what feels okay. This reconnects you with physical sensations trauma disconnected.

6. The Dialogue: Write conversations between your traumatized self and current self, between your critical voice and compassionate voice, between fear and courage, or between shame and truth. This helps integrate different parts of yourself.

Somatic Writing Exercise: Before you write, try this grounding technique: Place both feet flat on the floor. Take three deep breaths. Feel your body in the chair. Notice your hand holding the pen or touching the keyboard. This grounds you in the present moment before diving into difficult content, making the writing feel safer.

Write Therapy: A Step-by-Step Trauma Writing Process

Here's a structured approach for processing trauma through writing:

Step 1: Prepare Your Space - Find complete privacy, have tissues nearby, set a timer for 15–20 minutes, and have a plan for self-care afterward.

Step 2: Start With Safety - Write: "Right now I am safe. I am [age] years old. I am in [location]. What happened was in the past."

Step 3: Choose Your Focus - Pick one aspect: a specific memory, a feeling that's bothering you, a belief you want to challenge, or a part of your body that holds pain.

Step 4: Write Without Stopping - Let words flow without editing. If you get stuck, write about being stuck. If emotions arise, write about them. Keep your hand moving.

Step 5: Read and Respond - Read what you wrote (if you can). Then write what you notice about what you wrote, what surprised you, what you want to tell the person who wrote this, and one kind thing to yourself.

Step 6: Decide What to Do - You can keep it in a private journal, tear it up ceremonially, burn it safely, bury it, or keep some parts and destroy others.

Step 7: Transition Back - Do something grounding: wash your face with cool water, step outside, call a friend (you don't have to tell them why), do something creative, or move your body.

When Writing Feels Too Hard

Sometimes approaching trauma directly feels impossible. Try these gentler approaches:

Write Around It: Describe how your room looks when you're sad, write about a tree that survived a storm, create a character who's strong, or write about what safety feels like.

Use Prompts: Try "If my body could speak, it would say..." "The color of my pain is..." "I am learning that..." or "One day I will..."

Try Different Forms: Poetry, it doesn't have to rhyme, song lyrics don't have to sound like music, lists, drawing with words, or text messages to yourself.

Start Tiny: One word per day, one sentence, a haiku, or just the date and "I survived today."

Making Writing a Healing Practice

Create Rituals: Light a candle before writing, play specific music, write at the same time daily, or end with self-care.

Track Progress: Notice themes changing over time, celebrate small shifts, see your strength building, and watch shame losing power.

Be Patient: Some days words won't come, some days they'll overwhelm you. Both are okay. Progress isn't linear.

Stay Safe: Don't push too hard, take breaks, use your coping tools, and remember you're in control.

Your Voice Matters

Here's what I want you to know: Your words matter. Your story matters. Your pain matters. Your healing matters. Even if no one else ever reads a single word you write, the act of writing validates your experience and reclaims your voice.

You were silenced by abuse. Writing breaks that silence, even if only for you. Every word you write is an act of resistance against what happened. Every page is proof that you survived and are still here, still fighting, still healing.

Some days you'll write beautifully. Some days you'll barely scrawl a word. Both are victories. Both are healing. Both are you refusing to let trauma have the last word.

A Writing Promise

Start where you are. Write what you can. Trust the process, even when it's messy. Your words don't have to be perfect or profound. They just have to be yours.

The blank page is waiting—not to judge you, but to hold whatever you need to release. Your pen is not just a writing tool; it's a key to unlock what trauma tried to trap inside you.

Write your truth. Write your pain. Write your way home to yourself.

You've got this, one word at a time.

Where Were You God? A Conversation with the Divine

Many trauma survivors wrestle with profound questions about God's presence—or apparent absence—during their abuse. If faith is part of your journey, you might find yourself angry at God, doubting God's love, or wondering why you weren't protected. These feelings are valid and common.

If you're ready to explore these difficult questions through writing, this exercise offers a way to have an honest conversation with God about your trauma. If faith isn't part of your healing journey, feel free to skip this section.

For survivors wrestling with questions about God's presence during their abuse

Setup: Find a quiet space where you feel safe. Set a timer for 20-30 minutes if that helps you feel contained.

The Process: Start by writing your honest question to God. Don't worry about being "respectful" or "faithful" enough. God can handle your anger, confusion, and pain.

Write: "God, where were you when [describe your trauma briefly]?"

Then begin writing, expecting God to respond through your pen. You might think these are just your own thoughts, and that's okay. Don't stop writing. Let the words flow, even if they feel made up or uncertain. Write your doubts: "I'm not sure this is really you" or "How can I trust this?" Then keep writing, listening for what comes next.

Sample Conversation Starter: "God, where were you when I was being hurt? I've been told you're always with us, but I felt so alone.

I've been angry at you, and I don't know if that's okay. I need to understand..."

[Keep writing, letting whatever comes flow onto the page]

After Writing: Read what you've written. Notice any shifts in your understanding or feelings. You don't have to believe everything that came through your pen, but consider what might be true or healing for you.

The Transformation of Truth

What starts as pain on paper transforms over time: confusion becomes clarity, silence becomes voice, shame becomes self-compassion, isolation becomes connection (even if just with yourself), and powerlessness becomes agency.

Writing can take you from drowning in pain to swimming toward healing. Early pages might be full of rage and confusion. Later ones might contain wisdom, self-love, and even joy. The journey between them isn't easy, but every word is worth it.

Coaching Corner: The Page as Witness

When no one else saw what happened to you, when no one else validated your pain, the page becomes your witness. It doesn't judge, doesn't minimize, doesn't tell you to "get over it." It simply receives whatever you need to pour out. Every word you write is you saying, "This happened. This mattered. I matter." The page holds space for all the parts of your story—the ugly parts, the painful parts, the parts you can barely think about. And in that holding, something shifts. You're no longer alone with it. The page has seen, and somehow, that changes everything.

15

Creative Expression: Acting, Art, and Play

In the act of creation, we reclaim the power that trauma tried
to steal. Every stroke, every note, every movement is proof that
we are more than what happened to us.

REMEMBER WHEN YOU WERE little and could lose yourself in imagination? When you could be anyone, create anything, when play came naturally? Sexual abuse often steals that freedom, leaving you feeling like joy and creativity are things you don't deserve anymore. I know because I spent years believing fun was for "normal" people, not for someone carrying what I carried.

But here's what I've discovered: creativity isn't just for the untraumatized. In fact, it might be one of our most powerful healing tools. Acting, art, play—these aren't frivolous extras. They're ways to express what words can't capture, to feel powerful when trauma made you powerless, to rediscover joy when shame says you don't deserve it.

This chapter is about reclaiming your creative self, whether that's through drawing, drama, dance, or just letting yourself be playful again. You don't need talent. You don't need to share it with anyone. You just need to give yourself permission to create and play.

Why Creativity Heals Trauma

When trauma happens, especially sexual abuse, it attacks your sense of self. It makes you feel like an object, not a person. Like you don't have choices. Like your voice doesn't matter. Creative expression flips all of that.

You Become the Creator: You decide what to make, you control every choice, you express YOUR truth, and you reclaim agency.

Your Body Becomes a Tool, Not a Burden: Movement releases trapped trauma, creating engages your whole self, play reminds your body it can feel good, and art makes your hands instruments of healing, not shame.

You Process Without Words: Some things are too big for language. Art speaks what mouths can't. Movement expresses what stillness traps. Play releases what talking can't touch.

When survivors first try creating after abuse, they often just make angry scribbles or move without purpose. It isn't "art," but it's the first expression of feelings without words. That simple act of creation begins to crack open the numbness wrapped around you for protection.

Amara's Story: Finding Light Through Art

Let me share Amara's story to show how creativity can transform pain.

Amara's workplace harassment began when she was just 16 at her first part-time job at a local restaurant. Her manager, twice her age, would corner her in the walk-in cooler and make advances, using his authority to pressure her into compliance. When she finally quit, her parents were confused—it had been such good experience for a teenager.

At 18, she landed what seemed like a dream internship with a well-renowned marketing executive. But he was blatantly abusive in front of the entire office, commenting on her body and demanding she wear specific outfits that "enhanced her figure for client meetings." When she quit, her family was disappointed. He was a respected man in the industry—surely she could have handled a few inappropriate comments for such valuable experience.

Her next job at 19 seemed different. She was hired on the spot for a highly competitive position at a prestigious firm. Her family was thrilled—until the supervisor made it clear she'd been chosen for her appearance, not her qualifications. Despite knowing others were more qualified, she stayed longer this time, desperate to prove her worth through her work. But every day reinforced that she was decoration, not talent.

At twenty-three, after quitting her third job, Amara felt hollowed out. Each workplace had confirmed the same devastating message: her value lay in how she looked, not what she could accomplish. The pattern had convinced her that she was fundamentally worthless as a professional, hired only to be objectified. The shame was suffocating—she began to believe she must be inviting this treatment somehow. Her family's disappointment and friends' suggestions that she was being "picky" or "uppity" only deepened her self-doubt. Why keep trying when every opportunity seemed to reduce her to an object?

Then her roommate, Sarah, noticed her withdrawing—how Amara's shoulders curved inward like she was trying to disappear, how she spent weekends curled up on the couch instead of going out. Sarah gently encouraged her to join a community art class she'd found. "Just try it," she said. "No pressure. Just come sit with us."

Amara's first painting was pure rage—red and black slashes across white canvas, her hand moving like it had a mind of its own. She almost threw it away, embarrassed by the violence of it, but something about seeing her feelings outside her body felt relieving. The next week, she painted shadows—deep purples and grays that seemed to breathe on the canvas. Then a small figure huddled in a corner. Then that figure, slowly, standing up.

Color crept back in like dawn after the longest night. She started painting with yellows and blues, discovering she loved the way colors mixed into something entirely new, something that belonged only to her. Art class became her sanctuary—a place where her worth wasn't questioned.

The breakthrough came when the community theater needed volunteers to paint sets. Working on those backdrops, Amara found herself curious about the production itself. She started attending rehearsals, drawn to the way actors could become someone else entirely. One day, the director asked if she'd read lines for an absent actor.

Standing on that stage, pretending to be someone confident and valued for her talents, Amara felt powerful for the first time in years. Her voice, which had shrunk to whispers of self-doubt, grew stronger with each line. She auditioned for the next production and got a small part. Night after night, she practiced being strong, being seen for her abilities, using her voice to fill the theater. And slowly, that practice leaked into her real life, helping her remember she had value beyond what others wanted to take from her.

Amara's creativity didn't erase her trauma. But it gave her ways to express it, transform it, and eventually, transcend it.

The Many Faces of Creative Healing

Creative expression isn't one-size-fits-all. Explore different outlets and find what speaks to you.

Visual Arts: Drawing where even stick figures count, painting including finger painting which is therapeutic, collage by cutting and pasting images that speak to you, photography to capture beauty or truth, sculpting with clay to physically shape your experience, and digital art using apps to create.

Performance Arts: Acting to be someone else for a while, singing even just in your room, dancing as movement and expression, spoken word poetry, playing an instrument, and mime or physical theater.

Written Creative Arts: Poetry that doesn't have to rhyme, fiction writing to create the story you needed, songwriting, graphic novels or comics, and screenplays or scripts.

Play and Movement: Sports to experience your body as powerful rather than vulnerable, martial arts for reclaiming physical power, yoga for gentle reconnection with your body, building things like Legos, models, or crafts, video games which count as creative play, and improv games.

Creative Exercises for Trauma Survivors

1. The Feelings Color Wheel: Assign colors to feelings. When emotions arise, paint or draw with those colors. No need to make "things"—just let color express what you feel. You might paint black and red for anger, then slowly add purple for grief, blue for sadness, and eventually, yellow for hope.

2. The Mask Project: Create two masks (paper plates work)—Outside: How you show the world, and Inside: How you really feel. This validates that both exist and both are real.

3. The Power Pose Performance: In private, stand like someone powerful—a superhero, a queen, a warrior. Hold for thirty seconds. Speak one line they might say. Feel the difference in your body. This rewires your nervous system to remember strength.

4. The Safe Space Creation: Draw, build, or describe in detail a place where you feel completely safe. Add every detail—colors, sounds, smells, textures. This becomes a mental refuge you can visit anytime.

5. Movement Story: Put on music and let your body tell a story through movement. Start curled up if that feels right, then let your body show the journey—the hurt, the healing, the hope. No one needs to see this. It's just for you.

6. The Transformation Art: Take something "ugly" or broken and make art—paint on old newspapers, collage over magazines, decorate cardboard boxes, or make sculpture from recyclables. This mirrors transforming trauma into healing.

7. Character Creation: Invent a character who has the qualities you wish you had. Draw them, write about them, act like them for five minutes. This helps you try on strength, confidence, or joy in a safe way.

> **Somatic Creative Exercise:** Before creating, try this body awareness practice: Stand with feet hip-width apart. Shake your whole body gently for thirty seconds—hands, arms, shoulders, hips. Then stop and stand still, noticing the aliveness tingling through your body. This awakens creative energy and helps you feel present in your body before creating.

Working Through Creative Resistance

"But I'm not creative" is something trauma tells us. Here's the truth:

Every Human Is Creative: You were born creative. Trauma may have buried it. "Good" and "bad" don't apply here. Process matters more than product.

Start Ridiculously Small: Doodle for thirty seconds, hum one note, make up one dance move, write one word, or arrange objects on your desk.

Use Templates and Prompts: Adult coloring books, paint-by-numbers, dance along to videos, copy drawings you like, or use writing prompts.

Make It Private: Create in secret if needed, destroy it after if you want, use password-protected digital spaces. Remember: this is just for you.

The Playground Principle

Play isn't just for kids. After trauma, learning to play again is revolutionary. It says: I deserve joy, I can feel carefree, my body can be a source of fun, and I'm more than my trauma.

Ways to Play as an Adult: Video games (solo or with friends), board games or card games, sports (casually, no pressure), building with Legos or similar, puzzles (jigsaw, crossword, sudoku), silly phone apps, dance parties in your room, making up stories, and playing with pets.

Start with five minutes. That's it. Five minutes of letting yourself play without judgment.

Creating Community (When You're Ready)

While healing can start in private, eventually sharing creativity can be powerful: join drama groups (be someone else for a while), take an art class (structured creativity), join band or choir (creating harmony with others), try creative writing groups, participate in open mic nights, join online creative communities, and share anonymously at first if needed.

You don't have to share your trauma to share your creativity. Let people see your art, not necessarily your pain.

From Surviving to Thriving

Here's what changes when you embrace creativity after trauma:

Before: "I don't deserve joy." After: *"Joy is my birthright."*

Before: "My body is shameful." After: *"My body can create beauty."*

Before: "I have no voice." After: *"I express myself in many ways."*

Before: "I'm broken." After: *"I'm a work of art in progress."*

This transformation doesn't happen overnight. It's painted one brush-stroke at a time, performed one scene at a time, played one moment at a time.

The Creative Journey Back

Many survivors describe how trauma seems to steal their creative spark. The activities that once brought joy—whether drama, writing, art, or music—suddenly feel impossible or even wrong. Some quit their creative pursuits entirely, as if expressing joy would somehow minimize what happened to them.

But living without creative expression becomes its own form of suffering. When survivors begin to explore creativity again, they often start tentatively. Private sketches no one will see. Fragments of writing hidden away. Movement in the safety of solitude. These small acts of creation, however imperfect, become lifelines.

What many discover is that creativity offers what words cannot: a way to express the inexpressible. Through art, they can voice pain without speaking. Through movement, they reclaim agency over their bodies. Through any creative act—painting, music, building, designing—they begin to remember who they were before trauma and imagine who they might become.

This is why creative expression features so prominently in healing journeys. It's not about producing masterpieces or performing for others. It's about the radical act of creating in defiance of those who tried to diminish and silence. Every poem, every sketch, every dance, every song becomes a small victory—proof that the creative spirit, though wounded, refuses to be extinguished.

For many survivors, creativity transforms from something they used to do into something essential—a way to process, to heal, to celebrate still being here. In choosing to create, they choose life over mere survival.

Your Creative Revolution

You might think you're not creative. You might think fun is for other people. You might think trauma stole your ability to play and create. But that's trauma lying to you again.

Your creativity is still there, maybe buried under shame and pain, but intact. Every human has the capacity to create, to play, to express. Trauma might have dimmed that light, but it couldn't extinguish it.

Start today. Pick up a pen, a paintbrush, your body, your voice. Create something—anything. It doesn't have to be good. It doesn't have to make sense. It just has to be yours.

In a world that tried to make you powerless, creation is power. In a life where you were silenced, art is voice. In a body that holds trauma, play is revolution.

Create your way back to yourself. Play your way back to joy. You deserve both, and so much more.

The stage is yours. The canvas is waiting. Your story isn't over—this is just the beginning of a more colorful chapter.

Coaching Corner: Permission to Play

I want to give you something that trauma stole: permission. Permission to play without purpose. Permission to create without perfection. Permission to laugh without guilt. Permission to enjoy your body without shame. You don't need to earn joy through suffering. You don't need to be "healed enough" to deserve fun. Play isn't the reward at the end of healing—it's a tool for healing itself. So go ahead. Dance badly. Sing off-key. Paint outside the lines. The part of you that knows how to play? That's the part trauma couldn't touch. Let it out.

PART IV: REBUILDING RELATIONSHIPS

Creating Safety in Connection

16

Setting Boundaries: Learning to Say No

A boundary is not a wall that keeps love out. It's a gate that teaches love how to come in respectfully.

I F SAYING "NO" FEELS impossible, if you find yourself agreeing to things that make you uncomfortable, if you feel like your needs always come last—I get it. After sexual abuse, boundaries can feel like a foreign language you never learned to speak. The person who hurt me didn't just cross my boundaries; they taught me I didn't deserve to have any.

But here's what I've learned: boundaries aren't just nice to have—they're essential for healing. They're how you teach the world, and yourself, that you matter. That your comfort matters. That your "no" is a complete sentence.

This chapter is about learning to draw those lines, even when your hand shakes. It's about finding your "no" when trauma stole it. And it's about discovering that setting boundaries isn't selfish—it's survival.

Body Wisdom for Boundaries: Your body often knows before your mind when someone feels safe or unsafe. Learning to read these physical cues - tension, relaxation, gut feelings - is crucial for healthy boundaries. If you struggle to sense these signals, practice the body awareness exercises from Chapter 1.

What Boundaries Really Are (And Aren't)

Let's clear up some confusion. Boundaries aren't walls that keep everyone out, being mean or selfish, punishing others, or needing to explain or justify yourself.

Boundaries ARE knowing what feels okay and what doesn't, communicating your limits clearly, protecting your energy and wellbeing, teaching others how to treat you, and saying yes to yourself when you say no to others.

Think of boundaries like the walls of a house. They're not there to trap you inside—they're there to create a safe space where you choose who enters and how they treat your home. After abuse, you might feel like someone demolished your walls, leaving you exposed and vulnerable. But you can rebuild them, brick by brick.

Why Boundaries Feel Impossible After Abuse

Sexual abuse is, at its core, a massive boundary violation. Someone decided their wants mattered more than your safety, comfort, or consent. This teaches terrible lessons.

You Learn Your "No" Doesn't Matter: When someone ignores your boundaries—whether spoken or implied—your brain learns that saying no is pointless. Why waste energy on something that will be ignored anyway?

You Learn That Boundaries Equal Danger: Maybe setting a boundary led to punishment, anger, or worse abuse. Your nervous system remembers: boundaries = threat. So now, even thinking about saying "no" triggers your alarm system.

You Disconnect From Your Needs: To survive abuse, many of us learned to ignore what we wanted or needed. We became experts at reading what others wanted from us. This survival skill becomes a liability when you can't even identify what your boundaries should be.

You Feel Guilty for Having Needs: Abusers often make you feel responsible for their emotions or actions. This creates deep guilt around having any needs at all. Setting a boundary feels like you're being "bad" or "selfish."

These experiences layer on top of each other, teaching us that our boundaries don't matter, that having needs is dangerous, and that keeping others happy is more important than keeping ourselves safe.

Cameron's Story: Finding Their Voice

Cameron knew exactly when everything changed, but it didn't happen the way trauma stories usually unfold in movies.

It was Tuesday afternoon, 3:47 PM to be exact, and Cameron was standing in their kitchen making coffee when their phone buzzed with a text from their sister: "Mom's inviting Uncle Rick to Thanksgiving again. Just wanted to give you a heads up."

Cameron's hand froze halfway to the coffee maker. Uncle Rick. The family favorite who taught card tricks and remembered everyone's birthdays. The one who used to corner Cameron during family gatherings when they were younger, whose hands wandered where they shouldn't, who made everything feel like Cameron's fault for "being too sensitive" about "harmless affection."

But instead of the usual flood of panic, instead of the familiar spiral into self-blame and dread, Cameron felt something different: clarity. Not the desperate, drowning kind of clarity that comes with crisis, but the steady, grounded kind that comes after years of work.

"Not this time," Cameron said out loud to their empty apartment, the words surprising them with their firmness.

They'd been in therapy for eighteen months now. Not the kind where you lie on a couch and talk about your childhood for years, but practical, focused work with Dr. Martinez, who taught Cameron that boundaries weren't selfish and that their nervous system's reactions weren't character flaws. They'd practiced saying "no" in the mirror, worked through shame spirals with breathing techniques, and slowly rebuilt their relationship with their own instincts.

Cameron picked up their phone and typed back: "Thanks for the heads up. I won't be there if he is."

The response came quickly: "Come on, Cam. It's been years. Can't you just be civil? It's family."

There it was—the old script. The one that used to make Cameron fold immediately, apologizing for having feelings, minimizing their own experience to keep everyone else comfortable. Cameron could feel their chest tighten, the familiar urge to backtrack and people-please rising like muscle memory.

But they'd learned to recognize that feeling now. Dr. Martinez called it "the notification system"—their body's way of saying "pay attention, something isn't right here." Instead of ignoring it or pushing through it, Cameron paused. Breathed. Put their hand on their chest and felt their heartbeat, steady and strong.

They typed: "I understand that's hard to hear. I'm not trying to cause drama. I'm taking care of myself."

No explanation. No justification. No emotional labor to make their sister feel better about Cameron's boundaries. Just the truth, simple and clear.

The phone stayed quiet for twenty minutes. When it finally buzzed, the message was shorter: "I don't understand, but okay."

Cameron smiled—not because their sister understood, but because they'd discovered something powerful: they didn't need her to understand. They didn't need anyone's permission to protect themselves. The scared teenager who used to hide in bathrooms at family gatherings was still there, but they weren't driving anymore. Cameron was.

That evening, Cameron called their mom directly. Not to explain or defend or negotiate, but to inform: "I won't be at Thanksgiving if Uncle Rick is there. Would you like me to bring my famous stuffing to the Friday get-together instead?"

Their mom was quiet for a long moment. Then: "Your stuffing would be lovely on Friday, honey."

It wasn't the conversation Cameron had feared for years. There was no drama, no accusations, no family explosion. Just a mother who chose her child's wellbeing over a difficult conversation. It was, Cameron realized, exactly what they'd always hoped for but never dared to expect.

Later, lying in bed, Cameron thought about all the Thanksgivings they'd endured, all the family events where they'd smiled and played nice while dying inside. They thought about the teenage Cameron who believed their only choices were silence or family destruction. That Cameron couldn't have imagined this—setting a boundary that actually held, family members who respected it without understanding it, the possibility of protection without isolation.

Change hadn't come like a lightning strike. It came like sunrise—so gradually you don't notice until suddenly everything is illuminated.

The Building Blocks of Boundaries

1. Recognizing Your Limits: Before you can set boundaries, you need to know what they are. Pay attention to physical sensations (tension, nausea, wanting to run), emotional reactions (anger, resentment, anxiety), and thoughts like "I hate this" or "This isn't fair." These are your internal boundary alerts. Start noticing them without judgment.

2. Starting With Small Boundaries: You don't have to start with the biggest, scariest boundary. Practice with low-stakes situations like saying no to a food you don't like, asking for a few minutes before responding to a text, choosing what movie to watch, or saying "I need to think about it" instead of an immediate yes.

3. Using Your Body Language: Your body communicates boundaries too. Stand or sit up straight, make eye contact (if this feels comfortable), keep your voice steady and clear, use hand gestures that reinforce your words, and take up space—you deserve to exist fully.

4. Having Boundary Scripts Ready: When you're learning, having phrases ready helps: "I'm not comfortable with that," "That doesn't work for me," "I need some space," "Let me think about it and get back to you," "No, thank you," "I've decided not to," and "This isn't up for discussion."

Practical Boundary Exercises

The Mirror Practice: Every day, look yourself in the eye and practice saying "No," "I don't want to," "Stop," and "I'm not okay with that." Start quietly if you need to. Build up to firm and clear. This trains your voice to cooperate when you need it.

The Boundary Journal: Each day, write one boundary you wish you'd set, how it felt to not set it, what you could say next time, and one small boundary you'll practice tomorrow.

The Body Scan Check-In: Before agreeing to anything, pause and notice: Is my chest tight or open? Is my stomach calm or knotted? Do I feel expansive or shrinking? Your body knows. Learn its language.

The Broken Record Technique: When someone pushes past your no, repeat the same phrase. Them: "Come on, just this once." You: "I said no." Them: "But why not?" You: "I said no." Them: "You're being ridiculous." You: "I said no." You don't owe anyone an explanation.

The 24-Hour Rule: For bigger requests, always say: "Let me think about it and get back to you tomorrow." This gives you time to check in with yourself without pressure.

Somatic Boundary Exercise: Stand with feet hip-width apart. Extend your arms in front of you, palms facing out, as if pushing something away. Take a deep breath and as you exhale, firmly say "No" while pushing your hands forward. Feel the power in your body as you create physical space. This helps your nervous system connect the word "no" with the feeling of strength and protection.

Boundaries in Different Relationships

With Friends: You don't have to share everything, you can say no to plans, you can ask for support without fixing their problems, and you can have different boundaries with different friends.

With Family: You can love someone and still need boundaries. "Family" doesn't mean unlimited access to you. You can limit contact if needed, and you can refuse to discuss certain topics.

In Dating/Romantic Relationships: You set the pace for physical intimacy, you don't owe anyone access to your body. "No" is a complete sentence at ANY point. Past consent doesn't equal future consent, and you can change your mind at any time.

At School/Work: You can ask for help when overwhelmed, you can report inappropriate behavior, you can say no to extra responsibilities, and you can protect your personal time.

When People Don't Respect Your Boundaries

This is crucial: when someone repeatedly ignores your boundaries, they're telling you who they are. Believe them. You might hear "You're too sensitive," "I was just joking," "You didn't mind before," "You're being dramatic," or "I'm just trying to help."

These are manipulation tactics. Your boundaries are valid regardless of others' opinions about them.

Navigating Relationships After Trauma

Dating and friendships after abuse require extra care. Here's what to watch for:

Red Flags in Any Relationship: They push past your "no," they make you feel guilty for having boundaries, they move too fast (love bombing), they isolate you from others, they dismiss your feelings, and they test small boundaries to see what they can get away with.

Green Flags to Look For: They respect your "no" without questioning, they move at a pace that feels comfortable, they have their own boundaries, they communicate openly, they take responsibility for their actions, and they make you feel safe, not anxious.

Remember: you do not owe anyone your trauma story. You can have boundaries without explaining why. "I'm not comfortable with that" is enough.

The Boundary Ripple Effect

As you get better at boundaries, you'll notice several changes. People who respected you all along will support your new boundaries. People who benefited from your lack of boundaries will resist them. You will feel guilty at first—this is completely normal. You will have more energy for things that actually matter to you. You will start attracting healthier relationships. Most importantly, you will begin to trust yourself more.

A Personal Note on Boundaries

Learning boundaries after abuse felt like learning to walk again. Every "no" was terrifying. I was sure people would leave, that I'd be alone forever if I didn't keep everyone happy.

Some people did leave. And you know what? Good. They were people who only liked me when I had no needs, no limits, no self. The people who stayed? They celebrated my boundaries. They said things like "Good for you" and "I'm proud of you for speaking up."

Your boundaries are not mean. They are not selfish. They are not too much. They are the foundation of every healthy relationship you'll ever have—starting with the one with yourself.

Your Boundary Bill of Rights

YOU HAVE THE RIGHT TO SAY NO WITHOUT EXPLAINING

YOU HAVE THE RIGHT TO CHANGE YOUR MIND

YOU HAVE THE RIGHT TO PRIORITIZE YOUR SAFETY

YOU HAVE THE RIGHT TO YOUR FEELINGS

YOU HAVE THE RIGHT TO MAKE MISTAKES

YOU HAVE THE RIGHT TO BE INCONSISTENT AS YOU LEARN

YOU HAVE THE RIGHT TO PROTECT YOUR ENERGY

AND YOU HAVE THE RIGHT TO EXIST WITHOUT EARNING IT

Moving Forward

Start today. Pick one small boundary. Practice it in the mirror. Use it in real life. Notice how you feel. Then try another.

Your boundaries won't be perfect. You'll say yes when you mean no sometimes. You'll feel guilty. You'll wonder if you're being "too difficult." That's all part of the journey.

But with each boundary you set, you're telling yourself and the world: *I matter. My comfort matters. My safety matters. My voice matters.*

The person who hurt you tried to teach you otherwise. Every boundary you set proves them wrong. Every "no" you speak is a victory. Every limit you maintain is healing in action.

You couldn't protect yourself then. But you can now. One boundary at a time.

> **Coaching Corner: The Sacred No**
>
> Your "no" is sacred. It doesn't need justification, explanation, or apology. It stands complete, whole, and valid simply because you spoke it. Every time you say no to something that doesn't serve you, you say yes to your own worth. Every boundary you set is a love letter to yourself, saying "You matter enough to protect." The world taught you that your no was negotiable. Now you're teaching the world—and yourself—that it never was. Your no is your power returned to you. Use it liberally. Use it proudly. Use it knowing that each time you do, you're rewriting the story of what you deserve.

17

Finding Your People: Building Safe Relationships

Healing happens in connection. Not in the false safety of isolation, but in the brave vulnerability of letting safe people see the real you.

I F TRUSTING PEOPLE FEELS like trying to breathe underwater—impossible and terrifying—I hear you. After sexual abuse, especially when someone you trusted was the one who hurt you, the whole world can feel like enemy territory. I spent years believing that letting anyone close was just asking to be hurt again.

But here's what I've learned: isolation isn't protection—it's prison. And while not everyone is safe (that's real), safe people do exist. Learning to find them, trust them bit by bit, and let them see the real you? That's not just nice to have. It's essential for healing.

This chapter is about learning to spot safe people, building connections that actually help you heal, and doing it all at your own pace—without having to spill your whole story to anyone until (and unless) you're ready.

Why Trust Feels Impossible After Abuse

Sexual abuse is the ultimate betrayal. Whether it was a family member who should have protected you, a partner who claimed to love you, or someone in a position of authority—they taught you that trust equals danger. Your brain, being the excellent protector it is, filed that lesson under "NEVER FORGET."

Now your nervous system sees threat everywhere. That friendly coworker could be manipulating you. That neighbor who seems supportive might have an agenda. That person who likes you definitely wants something.

This isn't paranoia—it's protection. After someone you trusted crossed every boundary, after authority figures showed that power could be weaponized, your brain is doing its job: trying to keep you safe based on what it has learned.

The problem? This protective mechanism becomes a cage. It keeps out harm, yes, but it also keeps out connection, support, joy, and love. And humans aren't meant to heal in isolation.

What Makes Someone Safe?

Physical Safety Signals: Your nervous system constantly scans for safety or danger in relationships. This shows up in how your body feels - whether you feel relaxed or tense around someone, whether you naturally stand tall or find yourself hunching over, and whether your breathing feels normal or becomes shallow and quick. . The body awareness skills from Chapter 1 help you recognize these important signals.

Before we talk about finding safe people, let's be clear about what "safe" actually means:

Safe People: Safe people respect your boundaries without requiring explanation and don't push for information you're not ready to share. They make you feel calm in your body rather than anxious. Safe people are consistent in their words and actions and take responsibility when they mess up. They have their own boundaries, which is a huge green flag. Safe people don't make you feel like you need to perform or pretend to be someone you're not.

Safe People DO NOT: Safe people do not push past your "no" or make you feel guilty for having needs. They don't share your private information without permission or make everything about themselves. Safe people don't dismiss or minimize your feelings or make you feel like you're "too much" or "not enough." They also don't give you that sick feeling in your stomach that signals something is wrong.

Trust your body on this. If someone makes you feel tense, small, or on edge—even if you can't explain why—that's valuable information.

Liam's Story: Learning to Trust Again

Let me share Liam's journey to show how trust can slowly rebuild.

Liam was thirteen when his baseball coach began showing special interest in him. Coach K had an eye for talent, he told Liam's parents, and their son was exceptional—the kind of raw ability that could earn college scholarships, maybe even a shot at the pros with the right development. "He needs specialized training if he's going to reach his potential," the coach explained during a meeting that made Liam's parents beam with pride. "I only work with a select few players like this."

The private coaching sessions started innocently enough. Coach K would pull Liam aside after regular practice, praising his form and telling him he was different from the other kids—more dedicated, more naturally gifted. "You have what it takes to go all the way," he'd say, building up Liam's sense of being chosen, special, destined for greatness. The coach spoke of professional scouts, college recruiters, and the sacrifices necessary for elite athletes. "This is what separates the champions from everyone else," he'd explain when the training became more invasive, more personal. "If you want to make it to the big leagues, you have to trust me completely."

The abuse was packaged as mentorship, framed as the price of excellence. Coach K convinced Liam that what happened between them was part of the unique bond between elite athlete and coach—something ordinary players wouldn't understand. When Liam showed discomfort, the coach would remind him of his potential, of the scholarships at stake, of how disappointed his parents would be if he threw away this opportunity. The manipulation was masterful: Liam believed he needed this man to achieve his dreams, that walking away meant giving up everything he'd worked for.

The abuse shattered Liam's ability to trust his own judgment. If he couldn't recognize danger in someone his parents trusted, someone the whole community respected, someone who seemed genuinely invested in his future—how could he ever trust anyone again? The coach had seemed so safe, so caring, so legitimate. If that was all an act, then anyone could be acting. Anyone could be hiding ulterior motives behind kindness.

The betrayal also taught him that his value to others might always be conditional, transactional. The coach had claimed to care about Liam's potential, but really he'd just wanted access to Liam's body. This left him wondering: Did anyone care about him for who he was, or did everyone want something from him? The safest answer seemed to be to never find out.

By 26, Liam had built walls so high that no one could scale them. He'd left his hometown after college where everyone knew Coach K as a pillar of the community, where Liam would have to see his parents still speaking admiringly of the man who had "helped develop their son's talent." He couldn't maintain romantic relationships because intimacy required trust, and worked a remote job that allowed him to avoid most human contact. He pushed away college friends who tried to stay in touch, making excuses until they stopped calling. He became the person who ordered groceries online, lived alone in a studio apartment, invisible by choice. The loneliness was crushing, but it felt safer than risking betrayal again.

Then came his neighbor, Maria, a retired teacher with paint-stained fingers and a gentle laugh. She noticed Liam's isolation but didn't push. Instead, she'd leave homemade cookies outside his door with small notes: "In case you feel like having something sweet today." No pressure. No questions. Just an invitation he could choose to accept or ignore.

One day, Liam knocked on her door to return a plate. Maria was working on a watercolor landscape at her kitchen table, and they began talking—about art, about the neighborhood, about nothing important. She never pushed for more than Liam offered, never made him feel like his privacy was something that needed fixing.

This felt different. Safe. Like breathing after holding your breath for years.

Encouraged by this connection, Liam cautiously joined a community art class Maria had mentioned. There he met Jamie, who respected his need for space and never pushed for personal details. He also met Alex, who shared Liam's love of documentaries and could talk for hours about filmmaking without asking probing questions about Liam's past.

Slowly, carefully, Liam began to let people in—not all the way, not with his whole story, but enough to feel less alone. The walls didn't come down all at once. Some days he'd retreat again, declining invitations and hiding in his apartment. But each positive interaction taught his nervous system something new: not everyone who seems trustworthy is hiding something. Some people really are just... kind.

Building Trust: A Gradual Process

Start with Low-Stakes Connections: The barista who remembers your order, the librarian who recommends books, the neighbor you exchange pleasantries with, and online communities around your interests. These relationships let you practice being around people without deep vulnerability.

Use the Testing Method: Share something small and see how they handle it. Mention you're having a tough day (not why), share a minor preference or boundary, or talk about a hobby or interest. How do they respond? Do they respect your limits? Do they share appropriately in return? Do they remember what you told them?

Trust Your Gut Timeline: First meetings involve noticing your body's response. After a few interactions, do they remain consistent? Over time, do their actions match their words? Deeper connection only happens when and if it feels right. You don't owe anyone instant trust. Real friends will be patient with your pace.

Safe Relationship Building Exercises

1. The Safe Traits List: Write down qualities that make you feel safe, such as "Listens without interrupting," "Respects when I say no," "Doesn't gossip about others," and "Has their own life and interests." Look for these traits in people around you.

2. The Circle of Trust Visualization: Imagine circles around you—outer circle for acquaintances (coworkers, neighbors), middle circle for friendlier connections (hobby partners, group members), and inner circle for trusted people (may be empty at first—that's okay). You decide who moves between circles and when.

3. Boundary Testing Practice: Start with tiny boundaries like "I need to think about that," "I'm not a morning person," or "I don't like hugs." Notice who respects these without question.

4. The Energy Check: After spending time with someone, ask: Do I feel energized or drained? Do I feel more myself or less? Do I feel respected or dismissed? Your energy doesn't lie.

5. Safe Group Exploration: Join structured activities where connection has boundaries—art, fitness, or hobby groups; volunteer organizations; professional associations; or online communities for your interests. Shared activities create natural, pressure-free bonding.

Somatic Trust Exercise: When meeting someone for the first time, subtly place your hand on your chest or stomach. Notice: Does your body feel open or closed? Warm or cold? Expanded or contracted? Your body often knows before your mind does whether someone feels safe. Practice tuning into these physical signals—they're your built-in safety detector.

Recognizing Safe People: Green Flags

They Respect Your Pace: "No rush. Whenever you're ready." And they mean it.

They Have Their Own Boundaries: People who can say no are safer than people-pleasers.

They're Consistent: Their Tuesday behavior matches their Friday behavior.

They Validate Without Prying: "That sounds really hard" without demanding details.

They Share Appropriately: They open up too, creating balanced connection.

They Celebrate Your Growth: Your wins make them happy, not threatened.

They Handle Conflict Maturely: Disagreements happen without attacks or manipulation.

Red Flags in Any Relationship

Love Bombing: Excessive attention, gifts, or promises early on. Real connection builds slowly.

Boundary Pushing: "Just this once" or "If you really trusted me" are manipulation tactics.

Isolation Attempts: Making you feel guilty for other relationships or activities.

Inconsistency: Hot and cold behavior keeps you off-balance.

Victim Mentality: Everything is always someone else's fault. They take no responsibility.

Disrespecting Others: How they treat service workers, their ex, or their family is how they'll eventually treat you.

That Gut Feeling: Your stomach churns, you feel on edge, something feels "off"—trust that.

Special Note on Dating After Trauma

Romantic relationships can be especially triggering. Take it slow. You don't owe anyone physical intimacy. Past trauma disclosure is your choice, on your timeline. "No" is a complete sentence at any point. Your boundaries might be different than others'—that's okay. Safe partners will respect your pace without complaint.

Watch for Partners Who: Respect physical boundaries without sulking, don't pressure for trauma details, understand that trust builds slowly, have their own emotional intelligence, and make you feel safe, not anxious.

Building Your Support Network

You don't need twenty friends. You need a few safe connections: someone who makes you laugh, someone who listens without fixing, someone who shares your interests, someone who encourages your growth, and someone who sits with you in silence.

These might be different people, or one person might fill multiple roles. Quality over quantity, always.

When You're Ready to Share

If and when you decide to share your story, choose someone who's proven safe over time, start with general terms ("I went through something hard"), share only what feels comfortable, remember you can stop at any point, and know that their response tells you everything.

A Safe Person Will: Thank you for trusting them, follow your lead on how much to discuss, keep your story confidential, not make it about them, and check in without pushing.

The Healing Power of Safe Connection

Every safe relationship rewires your brain a little. Each respectful interaction teaches your nervous system that connection doesn't always equal danger. It's slow work, but it's powerful work.

After trauma, many survivors think they'll be alone forever. Trust feels too risky. But slowly, carefully, it's possible to find your people—the ones who prove through consistent action that they are safe. They don't heal you (that's your work), but they create a soft place to land while you heal yourself.

YOUR RELATIONSHIP BILL OF RIGHTS

YOU HAVE THE RIGHT TO TAKE THINGS SLOW

YOU HAVE THE RIGHT TO CHANGE YOUR MIND

YOU HAVE THE RIGHT TO DIFFERENT BOUNDARIES WITH DIFFERENT PEOPLE

YOU HAVE THE RIGHT TO END RELATIONSHIPS THAT DON'T FEEL SAFE

YOU HAVE THE RIGHT TO BE BELIEVED AND SUPPORTED

YOU HAVE THE RIGHT TO PRIVACY ABOUT YOUR TRAUMA

YOU HAVE THE RIGHT TO HEAL IN COMMUNITY

YOU HAVE THE RIGHT TO BE LOVED EXACTLY AS YOU ARE

Moving Forward in Connection

Finding safe people after abuse isn't about forgetting what happened or pretending everyone is trustworthy. It's about slowly, carefully learning to discern who deserves access to you.

Some people will prove unsafe—that's not your fault or a failure. It's information. Some people will surprise you with their kindness and consistency. Let them.

You weren't meant to heal alone. You weren't meant to carry this by yourself forever. Safe people exist, and you deserve to find them. One careful step at a time, one small trust at a time, you can build relationships that support your healing instead of threatening it.

Your trauma tried to convince you that you're safer alone. Prove it wrong. Not by trusting recklessly, but by trusting wisely. By choosing carefully. By letting safe people show you that connection can be healing instead of harmful.

You deserve a soft place to land. You deserve people who see you, respect you, and value you. They're out there, waiting to be found.

Trust yourself. You know more than you think you do.

Coaching Corner: The Gift of Discernment

Your trauma gave you something unexpected: the ability to read people deeply. You notice micro-expressions others miss. You feel energy shifts in a room. You sense danger before it announces itself. This hypervigilance that sometimes exhausts you? It's also a super-power. The key is learning when to listen to it and when to question it. Not everyone who makes you nervous is dangerous—sometimes your trauma is just loud. But that gut instinct that says "safe" or "unsafe"? That's real. Trust it. Use it. Let it guide you toward the people who deserve to know you. Your ability to discern safety isn't paranoia—it's wisdom earned through experience.

18

Moving Forward: Hope and Resilience

You are not what happened to you. You are what you choose to become in spite of it.

IF YOU'VE EVER THOUGHT "I'll never get past this" or "This is just who I am now"—I need you to know something. Those thoughts? They're trauma talking, not truth. I know because I lived in that hopeless place for years, convinced that what happened to me had stolen any chance at a real future.

But here's what I discovered: trauma might have changed your story, but it doesn't get to write your ending. Hope isn't about pretending everything's fine or forgetting what happened. It's about believing you can build something beautiful with the pieces you have left. And resilience? That's not about being tough or never struggling. It's about getting back up, even when getting up feels impossible.

This chapter is about finding that spark of possibility again, nurturing it into a flame, and discovering that you already have everything you need to move forward—even if you can't see it yet.

Understanding Hope After Trauma

Let's be real: hope can feel like a cruel joke after abuse. How can you hope for a better future when the past keeps dragging you backward? How can you believe in good things when someone taught you, viscerally, that the world isn't safe?

Here's what hope actually looks like for trauma survivors. Not "Everything will be perfect" but "Things can be different." Not "I'll forget this happened" but "This won't always hurt this much." Not "I'll be who I was before" but "I'll discover who I can become." Not "I'll never struggle" but "I'll learn to navigate the struggles."

Hope after trauma is gritty. It's realistic. It's choosing to believe in possibility even when your brain is screaming that you're stupid for trying.

Why Resilience Isn't What You Think

When people talk about resilience, they often mean "bouncing back" like nothing happened. That's not resilience—that's denial. Real resilience for trauma survivors looks different.

Getting Through, Not Getting Over: You don't have to "get over it." You just have to get through today. Then tomorrow. Then the next day.

Bending Without Breaking: Some days you'll feel strong. Some days you'll barely function. Both are resilience in action.

Creating Meaning from Pain: Not "everything happens for a reason" (ugh), but "I can choose what this means in my story."

Building on Survival Skills: You've already survived the worst. Those same skills can help you thrive.

You're already resilient. You're here, reading this, still fighting. That's proof.

Patrick's Story: Finding Light in Darkness

At twelve, Patrick's world shattered when a trusted neighbor began abusing him during weekend visits to help with small engine repairs. Mr. had offered to teach Patrick about fixing lawnmowers and leaf blowers—skills his single mother couldn't provide. But in the cluttered workshop that reeked of old motor oil and gasoline, the lessons became something else entirely.

Mr. C would start each inappropriate contact by framing it as educational. "This is how men bond when they're working together," he'd say, his voice casual and matter-of-fact. "It's normal—just something that happens between a mentor and student." When Patrick would stiffen or try to pull away, Mr. C would act confused and slightly hurt. "I'm just trying to help you become a man, Patrick. Your dad isn't around to teach you these things." He'd make Patrick feel ungrateful for resisting, like he was rejecting not just the touching but the entire mentorship. "I guess if you don't want to learn from me, I can find another kid who appreciates what I'm offering," he'd threaten, making Patrick feel like he was the problem for not understanding how "real learning" worked.

The trauma lodged itself deep in Patrick's nervous system. By 28, the smell of motor oil at gas stations would send his heart racing and make his vision tunnel. He'd have to leave immediately, hands shaking as he retreated to his car. His body carried the violation like a wound that never healed—muscles perpetually tense, always braced for danger that might not come but felt imminent. He'd abandoned his childhood dream of becoming a mechanical engineer after just one semester, unable to sit through labs where the industrial smells transported him back to that workshop. The freeze response that had trapped him as a child now trapped his entire future.

His body had learned that competence and skill made him a target. Being good with his hands, being teachable, being eager to learn—these qualities had attracted a predator. So Patrick made himself small, unremarkable, avoiding any situation where someone might notice his abilities or want to mentor him.

The turning point came during a community workshop on goal-setting at the local library. The facilitator said something that cut through Patrick's fog: "Write down your dreams, even if they feel impossible. Sometimes our dreams know things our logical minds haven't figured out yet."

Patrick stared at the blank page, pen heavy in his hand. Slowly, words came: "Build something that helps people. Work with my hands again. Feel proud instead of ashamed. Maybe teach kids so they know they can solve problems."

Seeing those words in his own handwriting awakened something. Maybe the person who wrote those dreams was still alive inside him.

He started small—volunteering for a community cleanup day, fixing broken playground equipment. When a child's bike chain came off and he instinctively knew how to repair it, he felt a flicker of his old self. Then he helped with a kids' robotics program, watching young faces light up when he showed them how gears worked together. Their excitement reminded him that his knowledge could help rather than make him vulnerable.

The biggest shift came when Patrick realized he wasn't trying to recover his twelve-year-old self. That boy was gone, and grieving him was necessary. But this Patrick—the one who survived, who chose to keep going, who found ways to help others learn—this Patrick was becoming someone remarkable too. Not the same, but not less than. Different, carrying both the wound and the wisdom that came from surviving it.

How Trauma Tries to Steal Your Future

Trauma is a thief, but not in the way you might think. It doesn't just steal your past—it tries to convince you it stole your future too.

"I'm too broken to have a good life" Trauma says: You're damaged goods. Truth says: *You are a survivor learning to thrive.*

"I'll never be normal" Trauma says: Normal is defined narrowly. Truth says: *There are many ways to be okay.*

"I don't deserve happiness" Trauma says: You're not worthy of good things. Truth says: *You deserve every good thing.*

"It's too late for me" Trauma says: You're stuck forever. Truth says: *It is never too late to start healing.*

"This is just who I am now" Trauma says: This damage is your identity. Truth says: *You are still becoming.*

These thoughts feel true because trauma is convincing. But feelings aren't facts.

Building Hope: Practical Strategies

1. The Future Letter: Write a letter from your future self (1 year, 5 years, whatever feels right) to current you. What would they say? What would they want you to know? This isn't magical thinking—it's possibility thinking.

2. The Evidence Collection: Keep a "proof of progress" list—got out of bed on a hard day, set a small boundary, tried something new, asked for help, made it through a trigger. These "small" wins are actually huge. Document them.

3. The One-Degree Shift: You don't need a complete life overhaul. Shift one degree. Instead of isolating all day, text one person. Instead of numbing with TV, try 5 minutes of journaling. Instead of saying "I can't," try "I am learning." Small shifts create new trajectories over time.

4. The Possibility Practice: Each day, notice one possibility—"I could try that new coffee shop," "I could learn to paint," "I could join that online support group." You don't have to do them. Just notice they exist.

5. The Resilience Inventory: List times you've survived hard things—the abuse itself, difficult days since then, moments you wanted to give up but didn't, times you asked for help, challenges you've faced. You have a track record of survival. Trust it.

Somatic Hope Exercise: Stand up and reach your arms toward the sky, spreading your fingers wide. Take a deep breath and imagine you're reaching for possibility, for future, for hope. As you exhale, bring your hands to your heart. Feel that hope settling into your body. This physical reaching and gathering helps your nervous system remember that the future exists and you can reach for it.

Growing Resilience: Active Practices

Physical Resilience: Physical resilience includes movement that feels good rather than punishing, sleep hygiene that honors your individual needs, nutrition approached as self-care rather than control, and seeking medical care as the support you deserve.

Emotional Resilience: Emotional resilience means feeling your feelings without drowning in them, developing self-soothing methods that don't cause harm, setting boundaries that protect your energy, and showing compassion for your own struggles.

Mental Resilience: Mental resilience involves challenging the lies that trauma tells you, learning new coping skills that serve you better, educating yourself about the healing process, and celebrating small victories along the way.

Social Resilience: Social resilience includes building safe connections with others, asking for help when you need it, contributing meaningfully to other people's lives, and finding your community of support.

Spiritual Resilience: Spiritual resilience means connecting to something larger than yourself such as nature, art, or purpose, creating meaning from your experiences, practicing gratitude for small things, and maintaining belief in the possibility of healing and growth.

The Hope Anchors

When hope feels impossible, anchor to these truths:

You've Survived 100% of Your Worst Days: That's a perfect track record.

Healing Isn't Linear: Bad days don't erase progress.

You're Not Alone: Millions of survivors are healing alongside you.

Growth Is Always Possible: Brains can change. Hearts can heal. Life can improve.

Your Story Isn't Over: You're still writing chapters.

Creating Your Vision

Not a perfect life, but a possible life. What would feeling safer look like? What would having support feel like? What would pursuing a dream involve? What would self-compassion change? What would hope make possible?

You don't need all the answers. Just willingness to imagine.

The Power of Small Steps

After trauma, massive change feels impossible. But small steps? Those are doable. Today: Take one full breath. This week: Try one new coping skill. This month: Connect with one safe person. This season: Notice what's slowly shifting. This year: Acknowledge how far you've come.

Hope isn't built in grand gestures. It's built in tiny, consistent choices to keep going.

The Journey to Hope: A Path Many Travel

When working with survivors, I often hear the question: "How can you be sure it gets better?" This question comes from a place I understand—not because I remember every detail of my own darkness, but because I've witnessed this same journey unfold in other lives.

For many survivors, hope feels dangerous—like extending a hand toward a flame that's already burned them. After experiencing how trust can be weaponized and power abused, optimism seems naive at best, self-destructive at worst. Why risk believing in better when disappointment feels inevitable?

But here's what I've observed: living without hope becomes its own form of suffering. The absence of light doesn't protect anyone—it just leaves them navigating in darkness.

The path forward often begins with almost laughably modest expectations. Not grand dreams of complete healing, but microscopic possibilities: finishing a meal without anxiety, reading a full chapter of a book, sleeping past 3 AM. These aren't the triumphant victories people imagine healing will bring, but they're real. They matter. They're the building blocks of recovery.

What continues to move me is how healing multiplies when shared. When survivors find someone who can hold space for their pain while gently suggesting that change is possible—this becomes sacred work. In witnessing another's courage, people often discover their own. In believing for others what they can't yet believe for themselves, faith in recovery strengthens.

This is why I'm passionate about this work: because I've seen people emerge from that hopeless place. I've learned that the way out isn't through pretending everything's fine, but through claiming one small light at a time until the darkness no longer owns them. While my own journey happened long ago, the privilege of walking alongside others keeps these truths fresh and real for me every day.

Your Resilience Toolkit

Build your personal resilience kit: songs that make you feel powerful, photos that remind you of good moments, quotes that speak truth to trauma's lies, activities that make you feel capable, people who believe in your future, small goals that feel achievable, coping skills for hard moments, and reminders of how far you've come.

This isn't toxic positivity. It's survival equipment.

The Truth About Moving Forward

Moving Forward Doesn't Mean: Forgetting what happened, pretending you're not affected, never having bad days, being grateful for trauma, or becoming who you were before.

Moving Forward DOES Mean: Carrying your story without drowning in it, acknowledging impact while building new life, having bad days and good days, creating meaning on your terms, and becoming who you're meant to be now.

A Final Note on Hope

You might not feel hopeful today. That's okay. Hope isn't a feeling you have to manufacture—it's a choice you make. A tiny choice to try one more day. To reach for one small tool. To believe that tomorrow might be different, even if today is hard.

You've already shown incredible resilience by surviving. By seeking help through this book. By refusing to let trauma have the final word. That's not nothing—that's everything.

Your future hasn't been stolen. It's been complicated, yes. Changed, absolutely. But it's still yours to shape. And you have more power than you know to shape it into something worth living for.

Start where you are. Use what you have. Do what you can. And trust that tiny steps forward are still movement. You don't have to see the whole path—just the next step.

Hope is waiting for you. Not the naive hope of "before," but the earned hope of a survivor who knows that darkness isn't forever. Who knows that they're stronger than they ever imagined. Who knows that moving forward is possible, one breath at a time.

You've got this. Not because it's easy, but because you're already doing it. Keep going.

Coaching Corner: Your Future Self Is Cheering

Close your eyes for a moment and imagine yourself five years from now. Not perfect, not "fixed," but further along this healing journey. That future you? They're looking back at current you with so much compassion and pride. They remember this moment—the doubt, the pain, the wondering if it gets better. And they're cheering you on, because they know what you can't yet see: you make it. You find your way. The path isn't straight and it isn't easy, but it leads to a life worth living. That future self isn't disappointed in your struggles. They're amazed by your courage to keep going despite them. Listen closely—can you hear them whispering? "Keep going. It's worth it. I'm proof."

PART V: DEEPER TRAUMA UNDERSTANDING

Advanced Concepts for Comprehensive Healing

19

Understanding ACEs (Adverse Childhood Experiences)

Your struggles make sense. Your body has been keeping score,
and now it's time to understand the game.

"THE CHILD MAY NOT remember, but the body never forgets."
When I first read those words from Dr. Bessel van der Kolk,
something clicked. All those "random" health issues survivors describe—the unexplained pain, the anxiety that seems to come from
nowhere, the way their bodies react to certain situations—it isn't random at all.

I've watched so many friends struggle with mysterious symptoms,
bouncing from doctor to doctor, being told it's "all in their head."
The chronic fatigue that no amount of sleep could fix. The digestive
issues that flared up during family visits. The autoimmune conditions
that seemed to appear after stressful anniversaries. Now I understand:
these weren't flaws or imagined problems—they were bodies keeping
score of wounds that had never been properly tended.

When I learned about how trauma lives in the body, so much clicked
into place. The way Jordan's shoulders would tense whenever someone
walked behind their chair. How Kia would get mysterious headaches

before certain social situations. The insomnia that plagued Riley during family gatherings—the anniversary reminders of their abuse.

If you've been wondering why you struggle with things that seem to come easily to others, why your body feels like it's constantly on alert, or why certain mental health challenges keep showing up—this chapter might connect some dots. The ACE Study revealed something groundbreaking: childhood trauma doesn't just affect our childhoods. It shapes our entire lives—unless we intervene.

But here's the important part: understanding your ACE score isn't about labeling yourself as damaged. It's about finally having an explanation for struggles you've probably blamed yourself for. And more importantly, it's about knowing that healing is possible.

What Are ACEs?

Adverse Childhood Experiences (ACEs) are potentially traumatic events that occur before age 18. The original ACE Study, conducted by Kaiser Permanente and the CDC, looked at ten specific categories: physical abuse, sexual abuse, emotional abuse, physical neglect, emotional neglect, household substance abuse, household mental illness, parental separation/divorce, incarcerated family member, and witnessing domestic violence.

The Missing Pieces

But here's what the original study missed: it was conducted primarily on white, middle-class participants. It didn't account for racism and discrimination, bullying, community violence, poverty, medical trauma, loss of a loved one, immigration trauma, or foster care.

Your "unofficial" ACE score might be higher than what this quiz captures. That matters too.

Why Your ACE Score Matters (And Why It Doesn't Define You)

The higher your ACE score, the higher your statistical risk for mental health challenges (depression, anxiety, PTSD), physical health issues (heart disease, diabetes, autoimmune conditions), substance use problems, relationship difficulties, and early death.

Scary? Yes. Destiny? Absolutely not.

Your ACE score explains risk, not certainty. It's like knowing you have a genetic predisposition to something—important information, but not a life sentence. What matters more than your score is what you do with the knowledge.

Taking the ACE Quiz

This quiz asks about experiences before age 18 and can bring up difficult feelings. You're in control here: take breaks if needed, skip it entirely if it feels too much today, have coping tools ready, and remember this is just information, not judgment.

1. Did a parent or adult in the household often or very often swear at you, insult you, put you down, or humiliate you? OR act in a way that made you afraid you might be physically hurt?

☐ Yes ☐ No

2. Did a parent or adult in the household often or very often push, grab, slap, or throw something at you? OR hit you so hard you had marks or were injured?

☐ Yes ☐ No

3. Did an adult or person at least 5 years older than you ever touch or fondle you in a sexual way? Have you touch their body in a sexual way? OR attempt or actually have oral, anal, or vaginal intercourse with you?

☐ Yes ☐ No

4. Did you often or very often feel that no one in your family loved you or thought you were special? OR your family didn't look out for each other or support each other?

☐ Yes ☐ No

5. Did you often or very often feel that you didn't have enough to eat, had to wear dirty clothes, or had no one to protect you? OR your parents were too drunk or high to take care of you?

☐ Yes ☐ No

6. Were your parents ever separated or divorced?

☐ Yes ☐ No

7. Was your mother or stepmother often pushed, grabbed, or slapped? Sometimes or often kicked, hit with a fist, or hit with something hard? OR ever repeatedly hit or threatened with a gun or knife?

☐ Yes ☐ No

8. Did you live with anyone who was a problem drinker, alcoholic, or used street drugs?

☐ Yes ☐ No

9. Was a household member depressed, mentally ill, or did anyone attempt suicide?

☐ Yes ☐ No

10. Did a household member go to prison?

☐ Yes ☐ No

Your ACE Score: _____ (Total number of "Yes" answers)

What Your Score Means (And Doesn't Mean)

ACE Score 0: You had fewer recognized adverse experiences. This doesn't mean life was perfect or that other challenges don't count.

ACE Score 1-3: You experienced some adversity. With support and coping tools, many people with these scores thrive.

ACE Score 4+: You experienced significant adversity. Higher scores correlate with more health risks, but remember: correlation isn't destiny.

Any Score: Your experiences matter. Your struggles are valid. Your healing is possible.

The Science Behind ACEs

When children experience trauma, their developing brains adapt for survival through constant stress response where your brain stays in fight, flight, or freeze mode. This includes disrupted development where brain areas for emotional regulation and executive function are affected. The body experiences an inflammatory response and stays in a state of inflammation. Trauma can even cause epigenetic changes that actually affect how your genes express themselves.

But here's the hope: brains are changeable. They can change. The same adaptability that allowed trauma to shape your brain allows healing to reshape it.

Beyond the Numbers: What ACEs Really Mean

Your ACE score is just the beginning of understanding. What also matters includes timing, which refers to when the ACEs occurred since earlier trauma often has deeper impact. Duration matters because there's a difference between a single incident and ongoing trauma. Severity is important because ACEs are measured as yes or no, but intensity matters significantly. Support makes a crucial difference, specifically whether you had any safe adults since one caring person can change everything. Other trauma refers to experiences not captured in the basic ACEs questionnaire. Protective factors are the elements that helped you survive and build resilience.

The Protective Factors That Matter

Research shows these factors can mitigate ACE impacts:

Individual: Resilience and coping skills, self-regulation abilities, sense of purpose, along with hope and optimism.

Relational: At least one safe, stable adult, peer support, safe romantic relationships, and connection to community.

Community: Safe neighborhoods, access to healthcare, educational opportunities, and cultural connections.

You might not have had these growing up, but you can build them now.

Understanding Your ACE Score Through a Healing Lens

Many survivors avoid taking the ACE quiz. Sometimes it's because they don't want to quantify their trauma. Other times, it's because deep down, they're afraid of what the number might reveal. But taking the quiz can be a powerful turning point.

A high ACE score can feel overwhelming at first—like a forecast of life-long struggle. It may stir fears of inevitable health problems, emotional patterns, or broken relationships. But here's the truth: your ACE score is not your destiny.

The science of trauma has advanced. We now understand neuroplasticity—the brain's ability to rewire itself—and the power of protective factors like supportive relationships, therapy, healthy lifestyle habits, and community. Post-traumatic growth is possible. Healing is possible.

Think of your ACE score like a risk factor—not a life sentence. Just as someone with a family history of heart disease might be more proactive about their diet and exercise, a person with a high ACE score may need to be more intentional about emotional regulation, stress management, and creating safety in relationships.

Your ACE score is a framework for compassion, not judgment. It's not about labeling you. It's about understanding what your nervous system has endured—and giving you tools to support it moving forward.

You are not broken. You are a survivor with new information. Now, you can use it to build a life that supports your healing.

Somatic Exercise for ACE Integration: After taking the quiz, stand up and shake your whole body gently for 30 seconds—hands, arms, legs, everything. This helps discharge any activation from remembering. Then place both hands on your heart and take three deep breaths, saying internally, "I survived all of this. I am here now. I am safe in this moment."

Using Your ACE Score for Healing

1. Practice Self-Compassion: Your struggles make sense. You're not weak, broken, or failing. You're responding normally to abnormal experiences.

2. Get Curious, Not Critical: Instead of "Why can't I just be normal?" try "What does my nervous system need to feel safe?"

3. Build Your Toolkit: High ACE scores mean you need more tools, not that tools won't work for you.

4. Prioritize Nervous System Regulation: Your body has been in survival mode. Teaching it safety is primary.

5. Seek Trauma-Informed Care: Whether it's therapy, medical care, or bodywork—find providers who understand trauma.

6. Create New Experiences: Your brain learned from adverse experiences. It can learn from positive ones too.

The ACEs You Can Give Yourself

Dr. Bruce Perry talks about "therapeutic ACEs"—positive experiences that can help heal. You can give these to yourself: attuned relationships, consistent safety, emotional validation, predictable routine, opportunities for success, and unconditional positive regard (from yourself!).

Rewriting Your Story

Your ACE score is part of your story, but it's not the whole story. It's the beginning chapters—the ones you didn't get to write. But you're holding the pen now.

Every time you make healing choices, you're writing new chapters. You choose a safe relationship over a familiar but harmful one. You practice self-care instead of self-harm. You speak kindly to yourself instead of repeating old criticisms. You ask for help instead of struggling alone. You create safety in your life. Each of these choices rewrites your story. You're creating experiences that contradict what your nervous system learned. You're proving that the past informs but doesn't control the future.

A Note on Family

Learning about ACEs can complicate feelings about family. You might feel anger at caregivers who didn't protect you, grief for the childhood you didn't have, guilt for "blaming" family, or confusion about loving people who hurt you.

All of these feelings are valid. Understanding ACEs isn't about blame—it's about clarity. Your caregivers likely had their own high ACE scores. Hurt people hurt people. This doesn't excuse harm, but it can help you understand it as part of a larger pattern you get to break.

Moving Forward

Your ACE score is not your destiny. It's your history. It explains why you've struggled, why certain things are harder for you, why your nervous system reacts the way it does. But it doesn't determine your future.

People with high ACE scores become healers, artists, teachers, and parents who break cycles. They build beautiful lives not in spite of their ACEs but informed by them. They develop superpowers like empathy, resilience, and the ability to help others.

Your ACEs required you to be extraordinary just to survive. Now you get to use that extraordinary capacity to thrive. It won't be easy. It might not be fair. But it's possible.

And you? You're already proof of that possibility. You survived. Now it's time to heal.

Resources

ACEs   Too High: acestoohigh.com

CDC   ACEs Information: cdc.gov/violenceprevention/aces

ACE   Interface: aceinterface.com

Remember: Your score is information, not identity. Use it as a map for healing, not a prediction of your future. You've already beaten the odds by surviving. Now let's see what else you can do.

Coaching Corner: Your ACEs Are Not Your Destiny

That number you just calculated? It's not a verdict. It's a map. A map that shows where you've been, not where you're going. Yes, the science is real—ACEs indicate increased risk. But you know what else is real? Neuroplasticity. Post-traumatic growth. The fierce resilience you've already shown by surviving to read these words. Your ACE score explains your struggles; it doesn't excuse you from healing, but it does give you permission to be gentle with yourself along the way. You're not broken—you're adapted for survival in a dangerous environment. Now it's time to adapt for thriving in safety. That's not just possible. For survivors like you, it's probable.

20

Sibling Sexual Abuse: The Hidden Trauma

Just because it happened in a home filled with love doesn't mean it wasn't abuse.

O F ALL THE SECRETS survivors carry, sibling sexual abuse might be the heaviest. It's the trauma that feels impossible to name, wrapped in so many layers of confusion, loyalty, and silence that many survivors don't even recognize it as abuse until years—sometimes decades—later.

If you're reading this chapter with your heart racing, if you're thinking "but we were just kids" or "but they're my sibling," I need you to know: what happened to you was real. It was abuse. And the confusion you feel about it doesn't make it less valid—it makes it more understandable.

This is the conversation no one wants to have. But you deserve to have it.

Why Sibling Abuse Stays Hidden

Sibling sexual abuse is actually more common than parental abuse, yet it's the least reported, least discussed, and least understood form of childhood sexual trauma. Here's why it remains hidden.

The "Kids Will Be Kids" Myth: Society often dismisses sibling sexual behavior as "exploration" or "playing doctor." But there's a clear difference between age-appropriate curiosity and abuse. Abuse involves power imbalance (physical, emotional, or intellectual), coercion or manipulation, secrecy and threats, repeated violations, and behavior beyond developmental norms.

The Equal Power Illusion: People assume siblings have equal power. They don't. Power differences exist in age (even 2-3 years matters), size and physical strength, personality (dominant vs. passive), parental favoritism, and social intelligence/manipulation skills.

The Family Protection Instinct: Naming sibling abuse threatens the entire family structure. It's easier for everyone—parents included—to minimize, deny, or reframe it as "normal."

The Unique Confusion of Sibling Abuse

This type of abuse creates specific kinds of confusion that make it especially difficult to recognize and heal from.

"But We Were Both Kids": Yes, you were. That doesn't make it okay. Children can abuse other children. If you were coerced, manipulated, or forced, it was abuse—regardless of your sibling's age.

"Sometimes I Initiated": Abuse creates confusing dynamics. If you sometimes sought the contact, it might be because it was normalized in your environment, you were seeking control in an uncontrollable situation, you were trauma-bonded, (an unhealthy emotional attachment formed through cycles of abuse and intermittent kindness) or you confused abuse with affection. This doesn't make you complicit. It makes you a child trying to make sense of something senseless.

"They Were Abused Too": Many sibling abusers were also being abused. This explains their behavior but doesn't excuse it. You can hold compassion for their pain while still acknowledging the harm they caused you.

"But I Love Them": You can love someone who hurt you. These feelings can coexist: love for the sibling you wanted, anger at the sibling who hurt you, grief for the relationship you should have had, and fear of the person they were or are.

The Many Faces of Sibling Abuse

Sibling sexual abuse isn't one thing. It can take many forms that are often minimized or misunderstood.

The "Game" That Wasn't: Framed as play but involved coercion, secrecy, or age-inappropriate sexual behavior. Ten-year-old Emma thought they were just "playing house" when her fourteen-year-old brother suggested they act out what "married people do." The play area was in the basement, dim even during the day. She remembers the weight of his body, the softness of the cushions and blankets he'd arranged on the floor as a "bed", and how his whispered "we're playing house" made her stomach feel hollow with something she couldn't name.

The Gradual Escalation: Started as seemingly innocent and slowly crossed boundaries until you didn't know how to stop it.

The Night Visits: Happened when parents were asleep or away, creating a terrorizing anticipation of darkness. The creak of her bedroom door became Lisa's warning signal. She learned to distinguish between her parents' careful footsteps checking on them and her older brother's deliberate silence as he slipped into her room. The digital clock's green glow would burn the time into her memory—11:47 PM, 12:23 AM, 1:15 AM—timestamps of terror that made her dread bedtime for years to come.

The Babysitter Scenario: Older sibling "in charge" used their temporary authority for abuse.

The Normalized Abuse: Presented as "this is what siblings do" or "this is how we show love in our family."

The Violent Abuse: Involved physical force, threats, or punishment for resistance.

The Emotional Aftermath

Sibling abuse creates unique emotional wounds that differ from other forms of sexual trauma.

Identity Confusion: Your first peer relationship was corrupted. This affects how you see yourself in relation to others.

Trust Devastation: If you can't trust family, who can you trust? This primal betrayal affects all future relationships.

Loyalty Conflicts: Especially intense if you're still in contact. Every family gathering becomes a minefield.

Shame Spiral: Often deeper than other abuse because of societal minimization and family denial.

Anger Complications: Rage at the sibling, parents who didn't protect you, and yourself for not stopping it.

Love/Hate Dynamics: The impossibility of cleanly hating someone you also have loving memories with.

Why Parents Don't/Didn't Protect

This is often the second betrayal. Parents might not believe you, saying things like "Your brother would never..." or "You must be remembering wrong..." They may minimize the abuse by claiming "Kids experiment" or "It wasn't that bad" or "You need to forgive and forget." Some parents blame you by asking "Why didn't you tell us sooner?" or "You should have stopped it." Others focus on protecting the family image with statements like "We don't talk about this outside the family." Sometimes parents feel overwhelmed and literally can't process the reality, so they shut down emotionally. Parents with their own trauma histories might normalize what happened because abuse seemed normal in their own childhoods.

This lack of protection often compounds the original trauma. You needed adults to keep you safe, and they failed—whether through ignorance, denial, or their own limitations.

Somatic Exercise for Sibling Abuse Survivors: This trauma often creates a feeling of being trapped in family dynamics. Stand with your back against a wall. Press your whole back firmly against it, feeling the support. Now step away from the wall and notice the space around you. Do this several times, feeling how you can choose closeness to support (the wall) or distance and freedom (stepping away). This helps your body remember you have choices now about proximity and boundaries.

The Right to Your Truth

Here's what I need you to know:

Your Experience Is Valid: It doesn't matter if others minimize it, if your sibling "doesn't remember," or if your family wants you to "move on." What matters is your truth and your healing.

You Don't Owe Anyone Silence: Family comfort doesn't trump your healing. You can speak your truth even if it disrupts dynamics. Your story belongs to you.

Boundaries Are Sacred: You can limit or end contact with the sibling, skip family events, refuse to pretend everything's fine, and protect your own children.

Forgiveness Is Your Choice (When You're Ready): Forgiveness is a gift you give yourself, not them. It doesn't mean reconciliation or continuing the relationship. The person doesn't need to know, be sorry, or even be alive. There's no timeline—you'll know when you're ready. Forgiveness can free you from carrying their poison, but rushing it or forcing it helps no one.

Navigating Current Relationships

If your abusive sibling is still in your life, you have options including no contact at all, contact only at large family gatherings, contact with specific boundaries, or limited, surface-level contact. Whatever feels safe for YOU.

At Family Gatherings: Bring a support person, have an exit strategy, stay in public spaces, limit alcohol (it lowers defenses), and plan self-care before and after.

If You Have Children: You are NOT obligated to give access. Trust your protective instincts. Don't leave them alone together. Your child's safety trumps family harmony.

Finding Your Voice

Speaking about sibling abuse is incredibly difficult. Consider starting with yourself by journaling about it, saying it out loud alone, and using the words: "I was sexually abused by my sibling." Tell one safe person like a therapist, trusted friend, support group member, or hotline counselor. When deciding about family, remember you don't have to tell them. If you do, have support ready, prepare for various reactions, and remember that their reaction doesn't change your truth.

The Complexity of Healing

Working with survivors of sibling abuse has shown me that the pain is always compounded by confusion and silence. The healing always begins with naming it clearly: *This was abuse. This was not your fault. This matters.*

If your family minimized it... If you were told to "get over it"... If you've been carrying this alone... If you still doubt whether it "counts"...

Let me be clear: It counts. You count. Your pain counts. Your healing counts.

Reflection Prompts

What would change if I fully believed this was abuse?

What do I need to grieve about the sibling relationship I didn't get?

How has this affected my other relationships?

What would supporting my younger self look like?

What boundaries would make me feel safer now?

The Path Forward

Healing from sibling abuse is possible, but it's a unique journey. Acknowledge the complexity—it's okay to have conflicting feelings. You don't need to sort them into neat categories. Find specialized support by looking for therapists who understand sibling abuse specifically. Many don't. Connect with other survivors—you're not alone. Support groups exist specifically for sibling abuse survivors. Define your own healing—maybe it includes confrontation, maybe it doesn't. Maybe it includes forgiveness, maybe it doesn't. Your healing, your rules. Break the cycle—many survivors become fierce protectors of children. Your vigilance can prevent future abuse.

A Final Word

Sibling sexual abuse thrives in silence and minimization. By reading this, by considering that your experience matters, you're already breaking those chains.

You deserved a sibling who was safe. You deserved parents who protected you. You deserved a childhood free from sexual trauma. The fact that you didn't get these things is not your fault—not even a little bit.

But you also deserve healing. You deserve to speak your truth. You deserve to set whatever boundaries keep you safe. You deserve to be believed and supported.

The little kid who was hurt by someone who should have been their playmate, their companion, their safe person—that kid deserves to be seen, heard, and fiercely protected by the adult you've become.

Your story matters. Your pain is real. And your healing is possible, one brave truth at a time.

Coaching Corner: The Sibling You Deserved

Close your eyes and imagine for a moment the sibling relationship you should have had. Maybe there's laughter without fear. Play without secrets. Disagreements without violations. Protection instead of predation. That imagined relationship? That's what you deserved. Grieving what you didn't get doesn't mean you're dwelling on the past—it means you're honoring the child who deserved safety and got betrayal instead. Let yourself feel that grief. It's not weakness; it's recognition of the profound loss that sibling abuse creates. And in that recognition, healing begins.

21

Betrayal, Trauma, and Not Being Believed

Sometimes the second wound cuts deeper than the first. Not being believed doesn't erase your truth—it reveals theirs.

T HERE'S A HORRIFIC KIND of devastation that comes with the moment you finally find the courage to speak your truth, and the person you tell looks you in the eye and says, 'That didn't happen.'

The Teaching of Two Arrows

There's an ancient Buddhist story that perfectly captures what happens when trauma survivors speak their truth and aren't believed. The Buddha once asked his student, "If a person is walking through the forest and gets struck by an arrow, is it painful?"

"Yes, teacher," the student replied.

"And if that same person is then struck by a second arrow, is it even more painful?"

"Of course," the student answered.

The Buddha nodded. "In life, we cannot always control the first arrow. However, the second arrow is our reaction to the first. This second arrow is optional."

He explained further: "When someone is struck by the first arrow, they feel pain—real, unavoidable physical pain. But the untrained person immediately begins to panic: 'Will I bleed to death? How will I get home? What will happen to my family?' They shoot themselves with a second arrow of mental anguish, turning their pain into suffering."

"But," the Buddha continued, "the wise person feels the pain of the first arrow and nothing more. They don't add layers of worry, self-blame, or despair. They tend to their wound and seek help, but they don't multiply their pain with their thoughts."

For trauma survivors, this teaching holds profound truth. The abuse—that's the first arrow. It hits, it hurts, and it's real. You had no control over that arrow being shot at you.

But when you finally find the courage to speak your truth and some-one looks you in the eye and says, "That didn't happen"—that's the second arrow. And unlike the first, this one is shot by another human being who had a choice. They could have believed you, sup-ported you, protected you. Instead, they chose to wound you again.

The cruel irony is that while you couldn't control the first arrow, others keep choosing to shoot the second one. And sometimes, that second arrow—the betrayal, the disbelief, the isolation—hurts even more than the first.

If the original abuse broke your body and spirit, not being believed broke something deeper—your trust in your own reality. This chapter is about that second wound, the one that sometimes hurts even more than the first. Because at least with the abuse, you knew it was wrong. But when someone doesn't believe you? You start to wonder if maybe you're the one who's wrong.

The Double Betrayal

Let me be clear about something: being sexually abused is traumatic. But being disbelieved, dismissed, or silenced when you finally speak up? That's what we call betrayal trauma, and it's its own special kind of devastating.

Dr. Jennifer Freyd coined this term to describe what happens when the people we depend on for survival are also the source of our harm—or when they fail to protect us from harm. It's not just about the bad thing that happened. It's about the people who were supposed to have your back and didn't.

Think about it: as children or young people, we're wired to need our caregivers. We need them for food, shelter, safety, love. So when they're the ones hurting us—or when they refuse to believe someone else is hurting us—our brains do this wild thing. They compartmentalize. They minimize. They literally help us "forget" or doubt our own experiences because the alternative (accepting that the people we need aren't safe) is too threatening to our survival.

Why Being Disbelieved Cuts So Deep

When someone doesn't believe you about your abuse, several devastating things happen simultaneously.

Your Reality Gets Questioned: Suddenly you're not just dealing with what happened—you're questioning if it happened. "Maybe I'm remembering it wrong?" "Maybe I'm being dramatic?" "Maybe it wasn't that bad?"

You Feel Crazy: Gaslighting doesn't just happen in romantic relationships. When a parent, sibling, or trusted adult tells you that your lived experience didn't happen, you start to feel like you can't trust your own mind.

The Shame Multiplies: First there was shame about the abuse. Now there's shame about speaking up. Shame about "causing problems." Shame about not being believed. It's shame layered on shame, and it's suffocating.

You Learn to Stay Silent: If speaking up led to more pain, your brain learns: keep quiet. This lesson can last decades, affecting every relationship you have.

You Feel Utterly Alone: Being disbelieved is profoundly isolating. If the people who are supposed to protect you won't even believe you, who will?

The Many Faces of Not Being Believed

Disbelief comes in many forms, and they all hurt.

Outright Denial: "That never happened." "You're lying." "How dare you say that about them." When Lacey finally told her mother about her stepfather's abuse, the silence stretched like a held breath in their sunny kitchen. The smell of coffee grew bitter as her mother's face hardened. "He would never," she said finally, her voice flat as newspaper. "You have such an imagination." The word 'imagination' hung in the air like a slap.

Minimization: "It wasn't that bad." "You're overreacting." "That's just how they show affection."

Deflection: "Why are you bringing this up now?" "You need to move on." "Let's not dwell on the past."

Victim-Blaming: "What were you wearing?" "Why didn't you tell me sooner?" "You must have misunderstood."

Selective Amnesia: They "forget" you told them. They never bring it up again. They act like the conversation never happened.

Choosing the Abuser: They continue relationships with your abuser. They invite them to family events. They post photos with them on social media.

Each of these responses sends the same message: your pain doesn't matter as much as our comfort.

Why People Don't Believe

Understanding why people don't believe doesn't excuse their betrayal, but it might help you stop blaming yourself. People don't believe for several reasons:

It's too painful. Believing you means accepting they failed to protect you—that's a guilt many parents can't face.

It threatens their world. If Uncle Darren is capable of abuse, what else don't they know? It's easier to decide you're wrong than to question everything.

They have their own trauma. Sometimes disbelief is intergenerational—they couldn't face their own abuse, so they can't face yours.

Reputation protection. "What will people think?" Often family reputation matters more than your truth.

Financial or social dependencies. If the abuser provides financial support or social status, believing you threatens their security.

Simple cowardice. Sometimes people just choose the easier path, and silencing you is easier than confronting abuse.

None of these reasons make their disbelief okay. You deserved to be believed, protected, and supported. Their failure to do so is about their limitations, not your truth.

What Not Being Believed Does to You

The effects of betrayal trauma run deep:

Chronic self-doubt. "Maybe I'm making too big a deal of this."

Difficulty trusting your own perceptions. You question what you saw, heard, or experienced.

Feeling like you need "perfect" evidence. You believe you must have ironclad proof to be believed.

Overexplaining or over justifying everything. You provide excessive detail to defend simple truths.

Difficulty trusting others. If those closest to you didn't believe you, who can you trust?

Feeling fundamentally unsupported. The world feels like an unsafe place where you're on your own.

Physical symptoms. Betrayal trauma literally makes you sick, often showing up as autoimmune issues.

These effects can last for years. You might find yourself gathering "evidence" before speaking any truth, as if preparing for cross-examination. That's what betrayal trauma does—it makes you defend your reality constantly.

> **Somatic Exercise for Reclaiming Your Truth:** Stand with your feet firmly planted, hip-width apart. Place one hand on your throat and one on your heart. Take a deep breath and as you exhale, say out loud (even if it's a whisper): "My truth is real." Feel the vibration of your voice under your hand. This is your truth, spoken by your voice, felt in your body. No one's disbelief can take that away.

Reclaiming Your Truth

Here's what I need you to know: just because someone shot that second arrow doesn't mean the first one didn't happen. Their choice to wound you again doesn't erase your original experience. Their comfort doesn't trump your truth.

Believe Yourself: This is the hardest and most important step. Even if no one else believes you, YOU can believe you. Your body remembers. Your nervous system remembers. Trust that knowing.

Find Your People: Not everyone will disbelieve you. There are people—therapists, support groups, friends—who will hear you and believe you without question. Find them.

Write Your Truth: Sometimes we need to see our story outside our heads. Write what happened. Write how it felt to not be believed. Make it real on paper.

Set Boundaries with Disbelievers: You don't owe anyone access to you. If someone chose not to believe you, you can choose to limit their place in your life.

Grieve What You Didn't Get: You deserved protection. You deserved belief. You deserved support. Grieve those losses—they're real.

If You're Not Ready to Tell

Maybe you're reading this and you've never told anyone because you're terrified of not being believed. That fear is valid. Here's what you can do: start with anonymous support (hotlines, online support groups), tell a therapist who specializes in trauma, test the waters with hypotheticals ("What would you do if..."), remember you don't have to tell anyone until you're ready, and know that your healing doesn't depend on others believing you.

A Message to Those Who Weren't Believed

I see you. I believe you. Your experience was real, regardless of who acknowledges it. Their disbelief is not a referendum on your truth—it's evidence of their inability to hold difficult realities.

You survived the abuse. You survived the disbelief. You're surviving still. That takes incredible strength, even when you don't feel strong.

The child or young person who spoke up and wasn't heard? They were brave. They deserved better. You can give them better now by believing them yourself, by surrounding yourself with people who believe you, by never again accepting relationships where your truth is negotiable.

Moving Forward After Betrayal

Healing from betrayal trauma is its own journey, separate from but connected to healing from the abuse itself. It requires several key elements:

Radical self-trust. You must learn to trust your own perceptions again, even when others question them.

Chosen family. Build relationships with people who believe and support you, even if they're not blood related.

Boundaries as self-care. Protect yourself from people who invalidate your experience.

Speaking your truth. Whether publicly or privately, continue to name what happened and how it affected you.

Integration. Accept that some people will never believe you. That's about them, not you.

The Power of Being Believed

When someone believes you—really believes you—it's like oxygen after drowning. It doesn't undo the betrayal, but it reminds you that support exists. That your truth matters. That you're not crazy.

If you've found even one person who believes you, hold onto that. Let it be evidence that more belief exists in the world. If you haven't found that person yet, keep looking. We're out here—survivors who believe other survivors, people who understand that children don't lie about abuse, humans who know that your truth is valid simply because it's yours.

Your Truth Stands

Whether or not anyone believes you, these things remain true: what happened to you was real, the pain you feel is valid, you deserved protection and didn't get it, you deserve healing and can have it, your truth doesn't require anyone else's validation, you are not crazy, dramatic, or wrong, and you are believed by many, even if not by those who should have believed you first.

Your story is yours. Your truth is yours. Your healing is yours. No one's disbelief can take those away.

The people who didn't believe you? They failed you. But you don't have to fail yourself. You can choose to believe your own experience, trust your own knowing, and build a life where your truth is honored—starting with how you honor it yourself.

That's not betrayal. That's recovery. That's power. That's yours.

Coaching Corner: Your Truth Is Your North Star

In a world that tried to make you doubt your own experience, your truth becomes your compass. It doesn't matter if they believed you. It doesn't matter if they still don't. What matters is that you know what happened. You know what you survived. You know what you've overcome. Let that knowing be your North Star—the fixed point you navigate by when everything else feels uncertain. Their disbelief is just noise. Your truth is the signal. Follow it home to yourself, where you've always been believed, where you've always been enough, where your story has always mattered. Because it does. And deep down, you know it.

22

Dissociation & Memory Gaps

Your mind's ability to leave when your body couldn't is not weakness—it's brilliance.

"**I** FEEL LIKE I'M watching my life through a foggy window."

"There are whole chunks of my childhood I just... can't remember."

"Sometimes I 'wake up' and realize I've been zoning out for who knows how long."

"I know something happened, but the details are like smoke—I can't grab them."

If any of these sound familiar, you're not losing your mind. You're not making things up. You're experiencing dissociation and memory gaps—two of the most common (and most misunderstood) responses to trauma.

Here's what I need you to understand right from the start: your brain did this to protect you. When reality became too painful, too overwhelming, too dangerous to fully experience, your magnificent brain found a way to help you survive. It's not weakness. It's not craziness. It's brilliance.

Reconnecting with Your Body: Dissociation often involves leaving your body mentally. The body awareness practices from Chapter 1 are essential tools for gently returning to your physical self. If you experience severe disconnection, the Expanded Body Inventory (Appendix B) offers step-by-step guidance for reconnection.

What Dissociation Really Is

Let's demystify this. Dissociation is your mind's emergency escape hatch. When things get too intense, your brain essentially says, "Nope, we're checking out for a bit," and creates distance between you and your experience.

It's like your consciousness has a dimmer switch. Sometimes it dims just a little (daydreaming during a boring class). Sometimes it dims a lot (feeling like you're floating outside your body). And sometimes, especially during trauma, it can shut off sections entirely (memory gaps).

Dissociation can look like spacing out—losing chunks of time, "coming to" somewhere without remembering how you got there. "It might show up as emotional numbness—feeling nothing when you 'should' feel something. Sometimes it's depersonalization—feeling disconnected from yourself, like you're not real. Or derealization—feeling like the world around you isn't real, like you're in a dream. Some survivors experience identity confusion, feeling like different "versions" of you exist.

Everyone dissociates sometimes. But trauma survivors often dissociate more frequently and more intensely, because their brains learned this was the best way to survive unbearable experiences.

The Part That Takes You Away

When you dissociate, it's not random—it's a protective part stepping in to shield you from overwhelming experience. This part learned, probably very young, that when reality becomes unbearable, the kindest thing to do is help you leave.

This dissociative part might pull you up and out of your body (like floating above), take you sideways into fog or numbness, help you time-travel to somewhere/somewhen else, or create walls between you and the present moment.

Understanding your dissociative protector means recognizing that this part is like an emergency evacuation specialist. When it senses danger (even if you're actually safe now), it pulls the fire alarm and gets you out. The problem is, this part might not have gotten the memo that the trauma is over.

When you notice dissociation starting, try communicating with your dissociative part. Thank this part: "I feel you trying to protect me." Orient to now: "We're in [current year], we're safe." Negotiate: "I need to stay present right now. Can you stay close but let me remain here?" Compromise: "If it gets too much, we can take a break."

Remember: The part that helps you dissociate saved you during trauma. Now it needs to learn new ways to help.

Why Your Memory Has Holes

Here's the thing about trauma memories—they don't get filed away like normal memories. When something traumatic happens, especially in childhood, your brain goes into survival mode. The part responsible for creating nice, neat, chronological memories? It goes offline.

Instead, trauma memories get stored in fragments: body sensations (that sick feeling when someone touches your shoulder), emotions (sudden panic for "no reason"), sensory flashes (the smell of cologne, the pattern on wallpaper), and behavioral responses (freezing when someone raises their voice).

These fragments are scattered like puzzle pieces throughout your nervous system. Some pieces might be crystal clear. Others might be completely missing. This isn't your brain failing—it's your brain protecting you from overwhelming content until you're ready to process it.

As trauma expert Janina Fisher explains, your brain essentially said, "This is too much to handle right now. Let's break it into manageable pieces and deal with it later." The problem is, "later" can be years or even decades afterward.

The Confusion This Creates

Living with dissociation and memory gaps can be profoundly disorienting.

"Did it really happen?" When memories are fragmented or missing, you might doubt your own experience. But body memories don't lie. If your body reacts to certain triggers, something happened.

"Why can't I just remember?" Because your brain is still protecting you. Memories often return when you're safe enough, supported enough, and resourced enough to handle them.

"Am I making this up?" No. The very fact that you're worried about making it up suggests you're not. People who fabricate stories don't usually question their validity this much.

"What's wrong with me?" Nothing. Your brain used a brilliant survival strategy. The fact that it's still using it just means you haven't fully internalized that you're safe now.

Living in the Fog: Understanding Your Experience

Many survivors describe their minds feeling like Swiss cheese—some memories painfully sharp, others missing entirely. They might recall the pattern on a shirt, the smell in the air, or the sound of a door closing... but not the year, their age, or what happened before or after.

This experience is common. It's not a sign of being "crazy" or broken—it's a sign that the brain did exactly what it needed to do to survive.

Jenny remembers the texture of the brown corduroy couch in vivid detail—how the ridges felt rough against her cheek, the musty smell of old fabric softener that never quite masked something else underneath. She can recall the sound of afternoon game shows playing in the background, the tick of the wall clock that seemed unnaturally loud. But ask her who else was in the room, what year it was, or how she got there? Complete blank. The memory is like a photograph with most of the image burned away, leaving only fragments that feel both intensely real and completely disconnected from time and space.

Dissociation is a trauma response. It's the brain's way of protecting someone when a situation feels too overwhelming or unsafe to fully process. For some, that means losing chunks of time or not being able to recall important life events. For others, it might look like "floating away" during difficult conversations, therapy sessions, or intimate moments—watching from above, going numb, or suddenly feeling sleepy or mentally blank when something hard comes up.

These aren't flaws. They're protective strategies.

The brain's message during trauma might have been: "This is too much. We need to leave now." And so, it did. And sometimes it still does—even years later, when it's no longer necessary.

Understanding this can be a huge relief. You're not losing your mind. You're living with a nervous system that learned to survive under extreme conditions. Dissociation and memory gaps are not failures—they're signs that your body and brain did their job. Now, healing involves helping your system learn: It's safe to stay. It's safe to remember. You're not in danger anymore.

Somatic Exercise for Grounding: When you notice yourself starting to dissociate, try this: Press your feet firmly into the floor. Cross your arms over your chest in a self-hug, with each hand on the opposite shoulder. Gently tap alternating shoulders—left, right, left, right—while saying internally, "I am here. I am now. I am safe." This bilateral stimulation helps integrate both sides of your brain and brings you back to the present.

Common Myths About Memory and Dissociation

"If you can't remember everything, it didn't happen" is a dangerous myth. The reality is that traumatic memories are often fragmented. Partial memories are still valid.

The idea that "real memories don't come back—they're always there" is also false. Trauma memories can be suppressed and resurface later when you're safer.

Many people think "dissociation means you have multiple personalities," but dissociation exists on a spectrum. Most people experience mild to moderate forms.

Some believe "you should push through dissociation," but dissociation is protective. Forcing through it can be retraumatizing.

The notion that "once you remember, you'll be fixed" ignores the truth that memory recovery is just one part of healing, not the destination.

Working with Dissociation (Not Against It)

The goal isn't to never dissociate again. It's to understand when and why it happens, and gradually expand your window of tolerance for staying present. Here's how:

Notice with curiosity, not judgment. "Oh, I'm starting to float away. I wonder what triggered that?"

Ground yourself gently. Press your feet into the floor. Hold something with texture (ice, a fuzzy blanket, a smooth stone). Name 5 things you can see, 4 you can hear, 3 you can touch. Smell something strong (peppermint, coffee, essential oils).

Track your patterns. Keep a simple log: When do you dissociate? What happens right before? This builds awareness without forcing change.

Expand your window slowly. Stay present for just one breath longer than comfortable. Then two. Baby steps.

Create dual awareness. "Part of me is floating away AND part of me is here in this chair." Both can be true.

When Memories Start Returning

If memories begin surfacing, here's what helps:

Don't rush. Your psyche is sharing what you're ready to handle. Trust the pace.

Write it down. Even fragments. Even if it doesn't make sense yet. Paper holds what your mind can't.

Find support. A trauma-informed therapist can help you process safely. You don't have to do this alone.

Validate yourself. "This feels real to me" is enough. You don't need proof or witnesses.

Care for your body. Returning memories can be physically exhausting. Rest, eat, move gently.

The Power of Not Remembering Everything

Here's something that took me years to understand: you don't need to remember everything to heal. Some survivors never recover full memories, and they still heal beautifully. What matters isn't having a complete narrative—it's having a compassionate relationship with yourself and your history.

Your body remembers what it needs to remember. Your mind reveals what you're ready to handle. The gaps? They're not failures. They're your psyche's way of saying, "This part isn't necessary for your healing right now."

Living with Compassion for Your Dissociative Parts

That spacey part of you? Thank it. It kept you alive. That forgetful part? It spared you from unbearable pain. That numb part? It helped you survive when feeling was too dangerous.

These aren't flaws to fix. They're protectors to appreciate. As you build safety in your life, they'll naturally relax their vigilance. Not because you forced them to, but because they finally believe the danger has passed.

A Note on Integration

Healing from dissociation doesn't mean you'll never space out again. It means you'll notice it happening more quickly, you'll understand why it's happening, you'll have tools to ground yourself, you'll be less frightened by it, and you'll have more choice about when to stay present.

Some days you'll dissociate more. Usually it means you're stressed, triggered, or approaching difficult material. That's okay. Your brain is saying, "We need to slow down." Listen to it.

You're Not Broken

If you recognize yourself in this chapter, please know: you're not broken. You're not crazy. You're not making things up. You're a survivor whose brain used every tool at its disposal to protect you.

The fact that you dissociate, that you have memory gaps, that sometimes you feel unreal—these are badges of survival, not signs of failure. Your brain loved you enough to spare you from the unbearable. Now it's learning, slowly, that you're strong enough to stay present.

Be patient with yourself. Be patient with your memories. Be patient with your dissociative parts. They're all part of you, and they're all welcome in your healing.

You don't need a perfect memory to have a valid experience. You don't need to never dissociate to be healing. You just need to keep showing up, as much as you can, with compassion for all the parts of you that survived—including the parts that survived by leaving.

That's not dissociation. That's dedication. That's courage. That's you.

Coaching Corner: The Wisdom of Leaving

Your ability to dissociate? That's not a flaw in your system—that's a feature. When a child cannot physically escape danger, the mind finds another way out. You learned to leave without leaving, to protect your essence when your body was trapped. Now, as you heal, you're not trying to lose this ability. You're learning when to use it and when you don't need it. The same wisdom that knew when to leave can learn when it's safe to stay. Trust that wisdom. It saved you then. It's still serving you now.

PART VI: NAVIGATING COMPLEX ISSUES

Addressing Specific Challenges

23

Sexuality, Boundaries, and Identity

Your sexuality was never broken. It was interrupted. And you get to decide what happens next.

L ET'S TALK ABOUT SOMETHING that might make you want to close this book: sex. Sexuality. Desire. Your relationship with your own body and with intimacy. I know—these topics can feel impossible to approach when your first experiences with anything sexual came through abuse.

But here's why we need to talk about it: sexual abuse doesn't just steal your innocence or violate your body. It hijacks your entire relationship with sexuality before you even get to discover what that relationship might have been. It's like someone scribbled all over the first pages of your story before you got to write them yourself.

This chapter is about recognizing that your sexuality—whatever it looks like now—belongs to you. Not to your abuser. Not to trauma. To you. And you get to reclaim it, redefine it, or completely reimagine it on your own terms.

Physical Intimacy and Body Awareness: Healthy sexuality requires connection with your own body first. If physical touch or intimacy triggers disconnection, work consistently with the body awareness practices from Chapter 1. The Expanded Body Inventory (Appendix B) includes gentle guidance for reconnecting with all parts of your body.

When Your Introduction to Sexuality Was Abuse

For many of us, sexual abuse was our first introduction to anything sexual. We didn't get to have awkward first crushes, innocent hand-holding, or figure out attraction at our own pace. Instead, we got violation packaged as "love," manipulation disguised as "special attention," or violence that taught us that sex equals pain.

This creates a particular kind of confusion. Is what I feel now real desire or trauma response? Am I attracted to this person or is this familiar dysfunction? Do I actually want this or am I following a script written by abuse? Is my lack of desire my authentic self or trauma numbing? Why does intimacy feel like danger even when I know I'm safe?

These questions can make you feel like you're navigating intimacy in a language you never properly learned, all the while trying to translate trauma into healthy sexuality. It's exhausting. It's confusing. And it's completely understandable.

The Boundary Confusion

If there's one thing sexual abuse destroys, it's boundaries. When someone crosses the ultimate boundary – the sovereignty of your own body – every other boundary becomes unclear.

You might find yourself unable to say no even when every cell in your body wants to. Or you might say no to everything because it's the only way to feel safe. You may not know what you actually want versus what you think you should want. Your body might not feel like it's really yours to make decisions about. You might believe that having boundaries makes you "difficult" or "broken."

Many survivors spend years having sex they don't want because they literally don't know they're allowed to say no. Not because anyone is forcing them anymore, but because early programming said that their wants didn't matter. Learning that you have the right to boundaries – and that real partners will respect them – can feel like learning to breathe for the first time.

The Identity Questions

Sexual abuse during childhood or adolescence doesn't just affect your behavior – it can shake your entire sense of who you are, especially regarding sexual orientation, gender identity, and your relationship with your body.

You might wonder: "Am I gay/straight/bi because that's who I am, or because of what happened?" "Does abuse 'turn' people gay?" (Spoiler: No, it doesn't) "What would my sexuality look like without trauma?" "Do I feel disconnected from my gender because of trauma?" "Am I exploring gender identity as authentic self-discovery or trauma response?" "How do I separate who I am from what happened to me?" "Why does my body feel like enemy territory?" "Can I ever feel at home in my own skin?" "How do I reclaim pleasure in a body that holds pain?"

These questions don't have simple answers. What matters is that you get to explore them without judgment, at your own pace, and with curiosity instead of shame.

The Many Faces of Trauma's Impact on Sexuality

Trauma affects everyone's sexuality differently. You might recognize yourself in one or more of these patterns:

Some survivors experience **hypersexuality** – using sex to feel powerful, valuable, or in control. Seeking intensity because nothing else feels real. Confusing sex with love because that's what you were taught.

Others experience **sexual avoidance** – complete shutdown of sexual desire, physical numbness during intimacy, panic at the thought of being vulnerable, avoiding relationships entirely.

Many **cycle between extremes** – periods of intense sexual activity followed by complete withdrawal. Wanting closeness but panicking when you get it. Craving intimacy but sabotaging it.

Dissociation during sex is common – floating away during intimate moments, watching from outside your body, and going through the motions without feeling present.

During intimate moments, Alex would find himself floating near the ceiling, watching his body go through the motions below. The warmth of skin, the whispered endearments, the gentle touch—all of it felt muffled, as if happening to someone else through thick glass. His partner would sometimes pause, searching his face. "Where did you go?" they'd ask softly, and Alex would struggle to find his way back down into his body, back into the moment that should have felt safe but somehow triggered every alarm his nervous system possessed.

Some survivors struggle with **confusion about consent** – not knowing how to say no, not knowing you're allowed to change your mind, feeling like you "owe" sex in relationships, or not recognizing your own desires.

Others find themselves drawn to **trauma reenactment** – being drawn to partners who remind you of your abuser, recreating abusive dynamics, or seeking familiar dysfunction over unfamiliar health.

None of these patterns make you broken. They're all normal responses to abnormal experiences.

When Pornography Becomes Complicated

For many survivors, pornography enters the picture as another layer of sexual confusion. Whether encountered accidentally as children, used as a way to understand sexuality after trauma, or turned to as a coping mechanism, pornography can create additional complications in an already complex healing journey.

Early exposure as trauma: Children who are exposed to pornography before they're developmentally ready often experience this as traumatic. The graphic sexual content can be overwhelming, confusing, and frightening to young minds not equipped to process what they're seeing. This early exposure can shape expectations about sexuality in ways that interfere with healthy development.

Brain reward pathway effects: Research suggests that pornography may affect brain reward pathways, particularly in developing brains. For trauma survivors who may already have disrupted stress and reward systems, this can create patterns of compulsive use that feel difficult to control.

Using pornography to "understand" sexuality: Many survivors turn to pornography trying to figure out what's "normal" sexually, especially when their introduction to sexuality was through abuse. But pornography often depicts the same dynamics that characterize sexual abuse – coercion, aggression, lack of genuine consent, and objectification – which can reinforce trauma responses rather than heal them.

Pornography as emotional numbing: Like other potentially addictive behaviors, pornography can become a way to escape overwhelming emotions, numb pain, or avoid dealing with trauma responses. The temporary relief it provides can create cycles of compulsive use followed by shame and disconnection.

Lauren's Story: When Boundaries Become Blurred

Lauren shares her story in her own words:

When Lauren was 16, she started going to a new youth group and met a boy a year older than her named Mitch. They started as friends, and hung out mostly in group and church settings. After a few months of friendship, they started going on dates, and she really liked the way they laughed together and how everything felt light and fun.

Almost immediately after they started dating however, Mitch began saying and doing things Lauren wasn't comfortable with, and asking her to reciprocate. Lauren said she wasn't interested in that, and wanted to wait before engaging in sexual activity. Mitch replied with things like "This is what couples do!" "I'm just really attracted to you, I have to do this." And "This is normal, we should do it too." Lauren didn't want to lose the fun they had before this started, and she wanted to be liked, and do what "real couples do." She didn't know how to balance what she wanted and what he wanted.

After saying "No" and "I don't want to do that," multiple times, she gave into Mitch's requests. Over the next year, the sexual acts got more and more intense, and Lauren became both more comfortable and uncomfortable with it. Many times she engaged or initiated physical contact. But often, she felt like she couldn't say no, or didn't know how to stop once they had started. It felt normal to progress with time, and she didn't know how to say "yes" one day and "no" the next.

If she did say she was uncomfortable with something, Mitch would say things like "I have to have this, or I will hurt myself" or "Sometimes I feel so depressed the only way I feel better is when we are physical." Lauren didn't know how to say no to that. She didn't want Mitch to hurt himself, she loved him and felt it was her job to help protect him. As the relationship progressed, so did the intensity and confusion Lauren felt. She felt stuck and unsure how to manage it. Eventually, it took the help of her family to get her out of the relationship.

After the relationship ended, she felt hollow and removed from herself. Things didn't feel normal. She turned to various coping mechanisms including pornography to make sense of what happened, and binge watching shows to numb out and remove herself from her thoughts. Her body felt weird; she thought "If he liked my body, and what he did was bad, does that make my body bad?" She felt small, and trapped where she was, scared of running into Mitch or his family in their small town.

Slowly, through finding hobbies and trying new things that inspired her to experience different places across the world, she discovered a path back to herself. Family and friends encouraged her to get to the root of her coping mechanisms, and to find resources to help her heal. She found books about healing, and a therapist that helped her uncover patterns and triggers in her life that were keeping her stuck.

Through therapy, Lauren learned to recognize how Mitch's emotional manipulation had made her question her own boundaries and instincts. She discovered that many of her coping mechanisms—including the pornography use, binge watching, and isolation—had been attempts to make sense of the trauma and numb the confusion she felt about what had happened to her.

Now, at 27 she can understand more clearly what actually happened to her, and recognize her triggers more easily. It's now easier to remind herself she is safe—she is here now, the danger was then. She no longer turns to dangerous and unhealthy coping mechanisms, and it's easier to turn to safer and healthier sources for coping.

Setting Boundaries with Sexual Content

If you find yourself in a complicated relationship with pornography, consider these questions:

How do I feel before, during, and after viewing sexual content? Am I choosing this consciously or using it compulsively? Does this content align with my values about intimacy and respect? Is this helping me understand healthy sexuality or keeping me confused? Am I using this to avoid dealing with difficult emotions or memories?

Setting boundaries might include:

Creating specific times and limits for any sexual content consumption.

Choosing content that depicts mutual respect and genuine consent.

Taking breaks from all sexual content to reconnect with your own desires.

Seeking support if use feels compulsive or is interfering with relationships.

Working with a therapist to understand the role pornography plays in your healing.

> **Somatic Exercise for Body Ownership:** Stand with your feet hip-width apart. Place your hands on your hips in a power pose. Take a deep breath and as you exhale, say out loud (or internally if that feels safer): "This is my body. I decide." Feel the strength in your stance. This simple practice helps your nervous system remember that you are in charge of your body now.

Reclaiming Sexual Autonomy

Here's the radical truth: you get to decide what healthy sexuality means for you. Not your trauma. Not society. Not even well-meaning partners. You.

This might mean celibacy while you heal. Or forever if that feels right. It could mean slow, careful exploration with trusted partners. You might seek professional support from sex-positive trauma-informed therapists. Some choose solo exploration to understand their own body. Others completely redefine what intimacy means to them.

Start with basic body autonomy. Practice small boundary settings: "I don't want to hug right now." "I need space." "Please ask before touching me." Start with low-stakes situations.

Learn what real consent looks like: enthusiastic, ongoing, reversible, specific. You can always change your mind. Always.

Do a body inventory. What kind of touch feels good? Safe? Triggering? Neutral? Map your body's responses without judgment.

Explore pleasure mapping. What brings you joy that isn't sexual? Start there. Build a relationship with pleasure that isn't complicated by trauma.

Clarify your values. What do YOU value in intimacy? Connection? Pleasure? Safety? Trust? Let your values, not your trauma, guide your choices.

Navigating Relationships and Dating

Dating after sexual trauma can feel like walking through a minefield blindfolded. Here's what helps:

Take it slow. You set the pace. Any partner worth having will respect that. If they push, they've shown you who they are.

Disclosure is your choice. You don't owe anyone your trauma story. Share if and when it feels right for you, not because you feel obligated.

Watch for green flags. They respect your boundaries without question. They check in about your comfort and consent. They handle "no" with grace. They make you feel safe, not anxious. They support your healing journey.

Trust your body. Your body knows. If someone makes you tense, anxious, or dissociative—even if they seem "nice"—trust that response.

Have a safety plan. Know you can stop anytime. Have your own transportation. Tell a friend where you are. Your safety matters more than politeness.

When Healing Feels Impossible

Some days, reclaiming your sexuality might feel hopeless. You might think you're too damaged for healthy relationships. You might believe you'll never enjoy sex. You might fear that no one will want you if they know your story. You might feel broken beyond repair.

These thoughts feel true but they aren't. Healing isn't about becoming someone who was never abused. It's about becoming someone who was abused and has reclaimed their power. It's about reclaiming your choices, your body, your pleasure, and your right to say yes and no.

A Personal Note: Reclaiming Your Sacred Sexuality

Reclaiming sexuality after abuse can feel like learning to walk again after an injury. What should feel natural may instead feel confusing,

even threatening. For many survivors, the path is marked by stum-
bles—choices made from pain, not from freedom. Moments where
intensity was mistaken for intimacy.

This doesn't mean you're broken. It means you're learning. Healing is
possible. With time, support, and kindness toward yourself, you can
begin to reconnect with your body—not as an object or a battleground,
but as your own. You can learn that your body is yours, your "yes" holds
meaning, your "no" is sacred, and pleasure is not shameful—it is your
birthright.

You do not need to be "over it." You do not need to be sexual to be whole.
What matters is that you know: your body, your boundaries, and your
identity were never meant to be stolen. They still belong to you. And if
you're ready, you can begin the journey to reclaim them.

Moving Forward

Your sexuality is not broken. It may be complicated, confused, or hiding, but it's not broken. It's yours. And you get to decide what to do with
it. Maybe that means taking sex completely off the table while you heal.
Maybe it means slowly, carefully exploring with someone safe. Maybe
it means redefining intimacy entirely. Maybe it means discovering that
asexuality is your authentic truth, not trauma response.

There's no right way to be a sexual being after trauma. There's only
your way. And that way is valid, whether it includes sex or doesn't,
whether it looks like what others expect or something entirely different. Your body is yours. Your boundaries are yours. Your identity
is yours. Your pleasure is yours. Your choices are yours. No one—not

even trauma—gets to take that away. That's not just recovery. That's revolution. And it starts with believing you deserve to write your own story, one choice at a time.

Your Bill of Sexual Rights

YOU HAVE THE RIGHT TO DEFINE YOUR OWN SEXUALITY

YOU HAVE THE RIGHT TO CHANGE YOUR MIND

YOU HAVE THE RIGHT TO SAY NO TO ANYTHING, ANYTIME

YOU HAVE THE RIGHT TO SAY YES ON YOUR TERMS

YOU HAVE THE RIGHT TO TAKE AS MUCH TIME AS YOU NEED

YOU HAVE THE RIGHT TO BE CELIBATE

YOU HAVE THE RIGHT TO BE SEXUAL

YOU HAVE THE RIGHT TO FEEL SAFE IN YOUR BODY

YOU HAVE THE RIGHT TO BOUNDARIES

YOU HAVE THE RIGHT TO PLEASURE

YOU HAVE THE RIGHT TO HEAL AT YOUR OWN PACE

Coaching Corner: Your Sacred Sovereignty

Your body belongs to you. Full stop. Not to your past, not to those who hurt you, not to anyone who thinks they have a say in what you do with it. After sexual abuse, reclaiming this basic truth can feel revolutionary—because it is. The person who violated you tried to make you believe your body was public property, that others could stake claims on it, that your boundaries were negotiable.

But here's what they couldn't steal: your inherent right to decide. Yes, they violated that right. Yes, they crossed boundaries that should have been sacred. But the right itself? That remains yours. Every choice you make now—whether to embrace sexuality or choose celibacy, whether to share touch or maintain distance, whether to explore pleasure or find peace in solitude—is you exercising your sovereignty. There's no "should" here. No timeline. No "normal" to achieve. There's only what feels authentic and safe for you.

Some survivors reclaim their bodies through intimate relationships. Others through solitude. Some through sensual pleasure. Others through athletic achievement or creative expression. All paths are valid. What matters is that YOU choose the path. Your body is not a democracy where everyone gets a vote. It's not a territory to be conquered. It's not a problem to be fixed. It's yours—wholly, completely, eternally yours.

If you're a person of faith, you may have learned that your body is God's temple (1 Corinthians 6:19). This beautiful truth was never meant to strip you of agency—it means your body is sacred and deserving of honor and protection. As the temple's appointed caretaker, you have both the right and responsibility to guard it, to set boundaries, to decide how it's treated. The person who abused you violated God's temple, which makes their sin even greater—but it doesn't diminish your authority as the one God entrusted with its care.

And that sovereignty? No one can take it from you again.

24

Inner Critic / Internalized Abuser

The cruelest voice in your head isn't yours. It's an echo of those who hurt you. You can choose to stop listening.

S URVIVORS OF SEXUAL ABUSE often carry internal messages shaped by moments of confusion, fear, or pain. These messages—sometimes loud, sometimes subtle—form an inner critic, a voice that repeats harmful narratives. This inner voice can sound convincing, but it's often rooted in trauma, not truth. Healing begins by recognizing these thoughts and choosing to speak to ourselves with compassion and clarity.

Inner Dialogue: From Trauma Voice to Truth Voice

Below are examples of how unresolved emotions might manifest in your thoughts, and healthier ways to respond. You are not the voice of your trauma. You are the one who can choose to respond differently.

The Voices and Their Truth

Fear says: "They won't like me unless I give them sex" or "I have to be sexual to be wanted." **Truth responds:** If someone doesn't like me without sex, they don't truly care about me. I deserve connection that honors me as a whole person.

Inadequacy says: "I can't be close to someone unless it's sexual" or "I don't know how to connect without being physical." **Truth responds:** Emotional intimacy doesn't require sex. Sharing dreams, values, and authentic conversation is real closeness too.

Shame says: "I'm bad because I liked it" or "I'm dirty and damaged because of what happened." **Truth responds:** What I felt was natural physical response. The abuser took advantage of that. I was a child—I'm not the one who should carry shame.

Low self-worth says: "I'm only good for one thing" or "My only value is what I can give physically." **Truth responds:** I am valuable and multi-dimensional. I bring intelligence, creativity, humor, and care to the world.

Fear of intimacy says: "I'll never let anyone close to me again" or "Everyone will hurt me if I trust them." **Truth responds:** My safety matters, and I can be cautious. But I won't let the abuser steal my capacity for healthy connection.

Guilt says: "It was my fault. I should have been stronger" or "I could have stopped it if I really wanted to." **Truth responds:** It was not my fault. I didn't deserve that, and I don't have to keep punishing myself. I choose healing.

Denial says: "I'm not angry. It wasn't that bad" or "I should just get over it and move on." **Truth responds:** What happened was serious, and it affected me. It's okay to feel angry. Acknowledging that helps me heal.

Hypervigilance says: "Everyone is dangerous" or "I can't trust anyone—they all want to use me." **Truth responds:** That person hurt me, but not everyone is the same. Healthy people exist, and I can learn to recognize them.

Somatic Exercise for Silencing the Critic

When you notice the inner critic getting loud, try this: Place one hand over your mouth and one over your heart. Take a deep breath. As you exhale, move the hand from your mouth outward, as if removing the critical words. Then press the hand on your heart gently, as if sealing in compassion. This physical gesture helps your body understand: the cruel words can leave, and the kindness can stay.

A Guided Reflection: Your Inner Voice Check-In

Use the following journaling prompts to gently explore your inner dialogue. Let this be a space of honesty and compassion:

What is a sentence I often hear in my mind about sex, love, or my worth? Where might that message have come from? If someone I loved said that about themselves, how would I respond? What would a caring, wise version of me say instead?

These thoughts do not define you. They are echoes of past hurt. You get to decide what voice you listen to now. You get to choose what's true.

Your Inner Critic as a Protective Part

That harsh voice in your head isn't the real you—it's a protective part that learned to keep you safe through criticism. This "manager part" often formed during abuse and took on the abuser's voice as a survival strategy. If you could criticize yourself first, maybe they wouldn't hurt you as much. If you kept yourself small, maybe you'd be less of a target.

Types of inner critic parts can include the Preemptive Striker, which says "I'll hurt us first so others can't." This part formed to beat others to the punch and needs to know we don't need to hurt ourselves to stay safe. The Perfectionist Protector declares "If we're perfect, we won't give them reasons." This part formed to prevent criticism through flawlessness and needs to know our worth isn't based on perfection. The Minimizer whispers "We're nothing, so expect nothing." This part formed to avoid disappointment and needs to know we're allowed to have needs and dreams. The Abuser's Echo repeats exactly what they said, formed by internalizing their voice, and needs to know their words were lies, not truth.

Like the Watchdog part we explored earlier that scans for danger, these inner critic parts developed as protective strategies during trauma. The Hypervigilant Scanner constantly evaluates threats and safety, while the Compartmentalizer helps manage overwhelming experiences by separating different aspects of our lives. Each of these parts, including the inner critic variations, served a purpose during trauma but may need gentle updating about our current safety and worth.

Befriending your inner critic means when you hear criticism, pause and ask: "What part is speaking?" Get curious: "How old is this part? When did it learn this job?" Thank it: "You've been trying to protect me." Update it: "The abuser is gone. We're safe now." Negotiate: "What if we tried encouragement instead?" Let your adult self lead: "I've got this now. You can rest."

Your inner critic doesn't need to be silenced—it needs a new job description. This protective part can become a discerning voice (not harsh), a boundary setter (not a wall builder), a growth encourager (not a perfectionist), and a wise advisor (not a cruel judge).

The Power of Challenging the Critic

Every time you challenge the inner critic, you're taking back mental territory that trauma claimed, practicing self-advocacy, rewiring neural pathways (that neuroplasticity from Chapter 8!), building a new internal relationship, and choosing healing over habit.

This isn't about positive thinking or denial. It's about accuracy. The critic lies. The truth heals.

Creating Your Truth Voice

Your truth voice might feel weak at first, especially compared to the critic's volume. That's okay. Like any muscle, it grows stronger with use.

Your truth voice speaks with compassion, not cruelty. It acknowledges pain without wallowing. It offers hope without minimizing difficulty. It sounds like someone who loves you. It focuses on growth, not perfection.

Ways to strengthen your truth voice include writing truth responses to common critical thoughts, recording yourself saying compassionate statements, borrowing the voice of someone who believes in you, practicing daily affirmations that feel believable, and celebrating small victories over the critic.

When the Critic Feels Like Protection

Sometimes we hold onto the inner critic because it feels safer than hope. If you expect nothing, you can't be disappointed. If you hate yourself first, no one else's hatred can surprise you. If you stay small, you won't be targeted.

But this "protection" is a prison. You deserve better than survival. You deserve an inner voice that champions your healing, celebrates your strength, and speaks truth to trauma's lies.

Cate realized she'd been having the same conversation with herself for twenty years. Every morning in the mirror, the voice would start: "Look at those bags under your eyes. No wonder nobody wants you. You're pathetic." The voice sounded so much like her stepfather that one day she actually gasped, covering her mouth as if the words had come from outside her body. That's when she understood: she'd been carrying his cruelty around like a ventriloquist's dummy, letting his voice speak through her own lips, letting his hatred masquerade as her thoughts.

Daily Practice: Catching and Correcting

Make it a practice to notice the critic. Pause when you feel bad about yourself. Ask: "What did I just think?" Identify: "That's the critic/trauma talking." Respond: "The truth is..." Breathe and let the truth settle.

This practice rewires your default mental pathways from criticism to compassion.

The Journey to Self-Compassion

Transforming your inner dialogue is not about perfection. You won't catch every critical thought. Some days the trauma voice will be louder. That's normal. What matters is the overall direction—toward kindness, toward truth, toward healing.

The critic might never disappear completely. But it can become just one voice among many, and not the loudest one. Your truth voice, your compassionate voice, your healing voice—these can become the chorus that drowns out trauma's solo.

A Final Note

The voice that tells you you're worthless, damaged, or only good for one thing? That's not your voice. That's the voice of those who hurt you, internalized and playing on repeat. But you're not a passive listener anymore. You're the DJ of your own mind. You get to choose what plays.

Choose truth. Choose compassion. Choose the voice that sounds like love.

Because that's what you deserve. That's what you've always deserved. And that's what you can give yourself, starting right now.

Coaching Corner: The Voice You Feed

There's an old Native American story about a grandfather teaching about the battle inside every person. "There are two wolves that live inside each of us, constantly fighting for control. The first wolf is full of negative emotions—anger that burns like fire, shame that whispers lies about your worth, fear that keeps you small, and harsh criticism that tears you down. This wolf feeds on pain and grows strong on self-doubt. The second wolf carries completely different energy—joy that lifts your spirit, peace that calms your mind, love that heals your heart, and compassion that speaks gently to your wounds. This wolf grows stronger when you treat yourself with kindness and choose hope over despair. Every day, these two wolves battle inside you. They're both hungry, both fighting to survive." He was asked, "But grandfather, which wolf wins?" The old man smiled and replied, "The one you feed." Your inner critic has been like that first wolf—well-fed by trauma, gorging on shame and fear for years. Every harsh word you've spoken to yourself, every cruel judgment you've accepted, every time you've chosen self-attack over self-compassion, you've been feeding the critical wolf until it became enormous and loud. But you control the food supply now. Every time you respond to criticism with truth, you're feeding the compassionate wolf. Every time you choose kindness over cruelty toward yourself, you're starving the critic. The critical wolf might howl as it weakens—that's normal. Let it protest. Keep feeding the voice that speaks love. In time, it will be the only one strong enough to be heard.

25

Self-Harm & Suicidality

Your pain is real. Your survival matters. And there are ways to
stay alive that don't require hurting yourself.

S ELF-HARM AND SUICIDALITY ARE among the most misunderstood responses to trauma. Especially for survivors of sexual abuse who
haven't disclosed their experience, these behaviors can feel like evidence of failure or brokenness. But they are not.

In trauma recovery, we now understand these are not acts of destruction, but often acts of desperation—our nervous system's last-ditch
effort to regain some form of control, relief, or even expression
when words feel impossible. Though it may sound counterintuitive,
self-harm can feel like the only way to stay alive—a way to convert
emotional pain into physical form, which can be felt, seen, and man-
aged.

For male survivors in particular, clinical research has emphasized how
important it is to shift from blame to understanding. According to
trauma-informed best practices, we should ask, "What happened to
you?" not "What's wrong with you?" This approach offers safety, trans-
parency, and choice—key elements of healing.

Trauma-Informed Principles for Understanding Self-Harm

Your behaviors developed to help you survive—they're not flaws in your character. When you get support, you should feel emotionally and physically safe. You deserve to have choices and control in every interaction with helpers. Asking for help shows strength, not weakness. The same inner strength that helped you survive can now help you heal.

Understanding Self-Harm as Communication

When we look at self-harm through a trauma-informed lens, we see it differently.

It's a language. When words fail, the body speaks. Self-harm might be saying: "My pain is real—look, here's proof," "I need to feel something other than numb," "This is the only control I have," or "External pain is easier than internal pain."

It's a coping strategy. Even though it's harmful, it serves important functions. It releases unbearable emotional pressure and provides temporary relief from emotional pain. It creates a sense of control when everything feels chaotic. It can break through dissociation when you feel numb or disconnected. Sometimes it communicates distress when you can't find words for the pain you're experiencing.

It's not about death. Often, self-harm is about trying to survive, not die. It's an attempt to manage life when it feels unmanageable.

A Note to Male Survivors

Many male survivors experience painful silence around their trauma. The weight of unspoken expectations settles heavy on their shoulders like an invisible coat they can never remove. You might feel: "I shouldn't need help; I should be strong," or "I'm alone in how I feel—other men don't talk about this."

Here's the truth: strength isn't about suffering in silence. Strength is reaching out when you're drowning. Strength is choosing to heal even when the world told you that "real men" don't have these struggles.

If you feel unsafe, dismissed, or ashamed reaching out, that says more about how trauma shaped your context—not your worth or potential for healing.

You deserve clear boundaries, transparent choice, and an invitation to be believed—even when the pain feels irrational or unbearable.

Somatic Exercise for Emotional Release: When the urge to self-harm rises, try this first: Fill a bowl with ice water. Take a deep breath and plunge your face into it for a few seconds. The shock to your system can provide similar relief to self-harm without the damage. Follow with gentle face drying and deep breathing. This gives your nervous system the intensity it's seeking in a safer way.

Body-Based Coping: When overwhelmed by suicidal thoughts or self-harm urges, grounding in your body can provide immediate relief. Use the emergency grounding techniques from Chapter 1.

Alternative Coping Strategies

When self-harm urges arise, try these alternatives:

For the need to feel: Hold ice cubes until they melt, snap a rubber band on your wrist, take a very cold or very hot (but safe) shower, do intense exercise for a few minutes, or eat something with a strong taste (sour candy, hot sauce).

For the need to see damage: Draw on yourself with red marker, paint on paper with red paint, rip up paper or cardboard, break ice cubes, or squeeze clay or Play-Doh.

For the need to release: Scream into a pillow, hit a punching bag or pillow, do jumping jacks or run in place, dance aggressively to loud music, or journal without censoring.

For the need to care for wounds: Draw "wounds" and bandage them, take care of someone else (a pet, a plant), create a self-care ritual, or tend to old scars with lotion.

Understanding Suicidal Thoughts

If you're having thoughts of ending your life, first: you are not weak, selfish, or crazy. You're in pain. Unbearable pain. And your brain is trying to solve the problem of that pain the only way it can think of.

Suicidal thoughts often mean several things. The pain feels bigger than your available resources. You want the pain to end, not necessarily your life. You need relief but can't see other options. Or your nervous system is completely overwhelmed.

These thoughts are symptoms, like a fever is a symptom. They signal that something needs attention, care, and support.

Safety Planning for Suicidal Thoughts

Create your safety plan. Write it out, and/or make a list on your phone and keep it near you.

Warning signs I notice: specific thoughts, feelings in my body, behaviors that signal I'm struggling.

Coping strategies I can use alone: distraction techniques, soothing activities, grounding exercises, reasons for living list.

People I can reach out to: friends who listen without judgment, family members who feel safe, online support communities, text lines: 741741 (Crisis Text Line).

Professional support: therapist's emergency contact, National Suicide Prevention Lifeline: 988, local crisis center number, hospital emergency room.

How to make my environment safe: remove or secure items that could cause harm, have someone hold medications, create physical safety.

My reasons for living: people I care about, goals I haven't achieved yet, experiences I want to have, pets who need me, curiosity about the future.

The Path from Surviving to Living

Self-harm and suicidal thoughts don't mean you're beyond help. They mean you're in survival mode, using the tools available to you. But there are other tools—safer tools—that can help you not just survive but eventually thrive.

Recovery doesn't mean you'll never struggle. It means you'll have more tools than just self-harm, you'll recognize warning signs earlier, you'll have people to reach out to, you'll know that feelings pass, and you'll have reasons to stay.

Breaking the Shame Cycle

Shame about self-harm or suicidal thoughts often makes them worse. Remember: these are common responses to trauma, many survivors struggle with these issues, it's not a sign of weakness, you deserve compassion not judgment, and healing is possible.

When to Seek Immediate Help

Go to an emergency room or call 911 if you have a specific plan to hurt yourself, you've gathered means to hurt yourself, you don't think you can keep yourself safe, or the urges are getting stronger despite coping attempts.

This isn't giving up or being weak. It's choosing life when your brain is telling you otherwise. That takes incredible strength.

Moving Forward

You do not need to punish yourself to express your pain. You can learn to listen to what your body and emotions are trying to tell you—with compassion and care. When you view self-harm or suicidal thoughts as messengers, not enemies, you reclaim your power.

This chapter is your invitation to begin reframing what's happening inside you. There is always a next step. There is always hope.

Even in your darkest moments, you are not alone. Other survivors have walked this path and found their way to light. You can too. One breath, one moment, one choice at a time.

Your pain is real. Your struggle is valid. And your life matters, even when—especially when—you can't feel it.

> **Coaching Corner: Your Survival Instinct Is Asking for Help**
> That part of you that self-harms or thinks about ending the pain? That's not your enemy. That's your survival instinct, desperately trying to help you the only way it knows how. It's saying, "This is too much. We need relief. We need change."
> Listen to the message, not just the method. Your survival instinct is right—you do need relief, you do need change. You just need safer ways to get there. Thank that part of you for trying so hard to help. Then gently show it the other tools available.
> Your survival instinct got you this far. Now let it learn new ways to keep you alive—ways that don't require hurting the body it's trying to save.

26

Safety Planning: Creating Space to Heal

Before you can rebuild, you need a place that feels safe to stand.

I F THERE'S ONE THING sexual abuse steals, it's your sense of safety. Not just physical safety—though that matters—but the deep, cellular knowing that you're okay in your own body, in your relationships, in the world.

That loss isn't just emotional. It's a full nervous system hijacking. The parts of your brain designed to keep you calm and grounded? They're stuck in alarm mode, constantly scanning for danger that may no longer exist.

Before diving into deep healing work, your nervous system needs to believe one fundamental thing: "I'm safe now." You might not feel it yet—and that's completely normal. This chapter will help you build safety step by step, starting exactly where you are.

Physical Safety Signals: Include body awareness in your safety planning. Learn to recognize early warning signs in your body - tension, shallow breathing, stomach knots - that indicate you need to use coping strategies. The body awareness exercises from Chapter 1 help you catch problems before they become crises.

What "Safety" Really Means

When we talk about safety in trauma recovery, we're talking about more than locked doors and avoiding dangerous people (though yes, those matter too). Real safety has layers:

Physical safety means your environment is secure. You know where to go and who to call if you feel threatened. Your basic needs are met.

Emotional safety means you can feel your feelings without punishment or shame. Your emotions are valid, even the "ugly" ones.

Relational safety means you have boundaries that people respect. You're not in relationships where you have to perform, pretend, or protect others from your truth.

Internal safety is the big one—beginning to feel safe inside your own skin, even when emotions rise, even when memories surface.

Building these layers takes time. You don't need them all perfectly in place to start healing. Even small increases in safety can make a huge difference.

Creating Nervous System Safety

Real safety planning for trauma survivors isn't just about avoiding dangerous people or situations. It's about creating conditions where your nervous system can finally relax.

When you've experienced trauma, your body gets stuck in a state of constant alert. Even when you're physically safe, your nervous system might still be scanning for threats, bracing for danger, or preparing to protect you. This is exhausting and makes healing nearly impossible.

Nervous system safety is about teaching your body that it's truly safe to let its guard down. Your nervous system—the network of nerves and brain circuits that control everything from your heartbeat to your stress responses—has been working overtime to protect you since your trauma. It's been your body's security system, constantly scanning for danger and keeping you ready to fight, flee, or freeze at a moment's notice.

This kind of safety operates on multiple levels—each one working together to signal to your brain and body that you can finally stop being on guard. When your nervous system receives consistent messages of safety from your environment, relationships, and internal dialogue, it can gradually shift from protection mode to healing mode. These different types of safety work like a team, each sending signals to your nervous system that say "it's okay to relax now" and "the danger has passed."

Environmental safety means creating spaces where your nervous system can settle. Look for environments where you can breathe fully and spaces that don't trigger hypervigilance or the need to constantly scan for exits. Create predictable routines that signal safety to your brain through consistency—when your nervous system knows what to expect, it doesn't have to stay on high alert for surprises. Choose sensory comfort with lighting, sounds, and textures that soothe rather than activate your nervous system. These environmental cues tell your body that this space is secure.

Relational safety provides your nervous system with social cues of security. This includes relationships where you don't have to perform or people-please—where you can be authentic without fear of abandonment or punishment. People respect your boundaries without making you feel guilty for having them. Support doesn't require you to be "grateful" or "fixed" in return. These relationships signal to your nervous system that you're valued and protected, not threatened.

Personal permission gives your nervous system relief from internal pressure. This means permission to say no without explanation—your "no" is complete and doesn't require justification. You can feel your feelings without judgment, having room to be sad, angry, scared, or numb without someone trying to fix or minimize your experience. You can rest without feeling guilty, understanding that rest is healing, not laziness. This self-permission tells your nervous system it's safe to be human.

Internal safety creates peace within your own mind. This includes permission to have needs—wanting comfort, support, or space is human, not selfish. You have freedom from internal criticism, learning to speak to yourself with the kindness you'd show a friend. You can trust in your own perceptions, believing your instincts and experiences are valid. This internal kindness signals to your nervous system that even your own thoughts are a safe place to be.

Physical safety keeps your body alive. Nervous system safety lets your body heal.

When your nervous system feels safe, several things become possible. Your body can actually relax instead of staying perpetually tense. Your sleep improves because your brain isn't keeping watch all night. Your emotions become more manageable because you're not constantly flooded with stress hormones. Your capacity for joy, connection, and creativity returns. Decision-making becomes clearer because you're not operating from survival mode.

The goal isn't to create a perfectly safe world—that's impossible. The goal is to create enough safety that your nervous system can shift from "survive" to "heal."

The goal isn't to create a perfectly safe world—that's impossible. The goal is to create enough safety that your nervous system can shift from "survive" to "heal."

Creating Your Safety Plan

A safety plan isn't just for crisis moments (though it helps then too). It's an act of radical self-respect—a way of telling your nervous system: "I matter. I deserve to feel okay. I'm worth protecting."

Let's build your plan together, piece by piece.

1. Daily Grounding Anchors

Your nervous system needs regular reminders that the danger has passed. Create small rituals throughout your day.

A morning reset might include simple stretches to reconnect with your body, three deep breaths before getting out of bed, a phrase like "I'm safe in this moment," and lighting a candle or opening curtains—something that says "new day."

Throughout the day, use phone reminders with grounding messages, scheduled body check-ins asking "What do I need right now?" and transition rituals between activities. These rituals might include taking three deep breaths, doing a gentle stretch, or repeating an affirmation before moving from one task to the next.

Evening wind-down could include dimming lights to signal safety, gentle movement or stretching, writing three things that went okay today, and creating a ritual that signals the day is finished and you can rest. This might be changing into comfortable clothes, saying "I did enough today," or having a consistent sleep routine that tells your nervous system it's time to let go of the day's vigilance.

Create Your Daily Grounding Card: List 3-5 things that reliably calm you: a specific song, a texture like a soft blanket or smooth stone, a scent such as lavender or coffee, a movement like stretching or walking, or a phrase that soothes you. Keep this list accessible—on your phone, in your wallet, or taped to your mirror.

Somatic Safety Exercise: Create a "safety sandwich" with your body. Lie down and place one heavy blanket under you and another on top (weighted blankets work great). Feel the pressure from above and support from below. Breathe deeply and let your body register: "I am held. I am contained. I am safe." This bilateral pressure calms the nervous system and creates a felt sense of security.

2. Emergency Response Plan

Sometimes trauma responses spike without warning. When you're triggered, thinking clearly becomes nearly impossible. That's why you need a plan created when you're calm.

Your emergency toolkit includes a safe people list: Who can you text when you're struggling? Who can sit with you without trying to fix? Who respects your boundaries? Include hotline numbers: RAINN (1-800-656-4673).

Identify safe spaces. Where can you go to feel secure? This might be a friend's house, the library, a coffee shop, or even your car. What makes a space feel safe to you? How can you make your current space safer?

Gather grounding tools: Keep physical items that help you feel grounded and present. These might include ice packs or cold water for temperature grounding, a soft blanket or stuffed animal for comfort, essential oils or strong mints for scent grounding, fidget tools or a stress ball for tactile support, and a playlist of calming music for auditory soothing.

Develop communication strategies: Create simple ways to ask for help when words feel hard. Establish code words with trusted people such as "I'm having a hard time." Prepare pre-written texts you can send when speaking feels impossible, like "Triggered. Need support. No questions please." Practice boundary phrases you can use when you need space, such as "I need space right now."

3. Your Personal Safety Assessment

Take inventory of where you feel safe and where you don't:

Life Area	Safety Level (1-10)	What Helps	What Hurts	One Small Change
Home/Living Space				
Work/School				
Close Relationships				
Body/Physical Self				
Online Spaces				
Internal World				

This isn't about achieving perfect safety everywhere. It's about awareness and small improvements.

4. Boundary Planning

Boundaries aren't walls—they're gates. They help you decide what's safe to let in and what needs to stay out.

Boundary planning questions: What behaviors make me feel unsafe? What do I need to feel more secure? How will I communicate this boundary? What will I do if someone crosses it? Who in my life respects my boundaries?

Practice phrases: "I need to think about that," "That doesn't work for me," "I'm not comfortable with that," "Let's find another way."

5. Sleep Safety Plan

Nighttime can be especially challenging for survivors. Your defenses are down, the world is quiet, and your mind might wander to dark places.

Creating nighttime safety includes several elements. Establish a consistent bedtime routine—your brain loves predictability. Limit screens 30 minutes before bed. Use a white noise or calming sounds. Keep a nightlight if darkness triggers you. Try a weighted blanket for grounding. Keep a journal beside your bed for worried thoughts. Practice safe imagery by imagining a protective place.

If you wake up triggered: Remind yourself: "I'm safe. It's [current year]. I'm in my room." Use grounding techniques. Have water nearby. Keep a comfort object close.

6. Internal Safety Phrases

When your inner world feels chaotic, these phrases can anchor you: "This feeling is temporary," "I'm having a trauma response, but I'm safe now," "My feelings are valid, but they're not facts," "I can ask for help," "I've survived before, I can survive this," and "This will pass."

Building Your Support Network

Safety isn't just about solo strategies—it's about having people who've got your back:

Inner circle: 1-2 people who know your story and can handle crisis moments.

Middle circle: Friends who support you without needing details.

Outer circle: Acquaintances who contribute positivity to your life.

Professional support: Therapist, coach, or counselor who understands trauma.

Making Your Environment Safer

Small changes can make a big difference: rearrange furniture so you can see the door, add locks that make you feel secure, remove or store triggering items, create a "safe corner" with comforting objects, use lighting that feels good, add plants or art that soothes you.

The Digital Safety Plan

Online spaces need boundaries too: curate your social media feeds, block accounts that trigger you, set time limits on apps, create separate emails for different life areas, use privacy settings liberally, and have a plan for when you encounter triggers online.

Safety Is a Practice, Not Perfection

Building safety isn't a one-time event. It's an ongoing practice that evolves as you heal. Some days you'll feel safer than others. That's normal. What matters is that you keep choosing to prioritize your well-being.

You don't have to earn safety by being "healed enough" or "stable enough." You deserve safety right now, exactly as you are. Every small step toward feeling safer is an act of rebellion against what trauma taught you.

You Already Deserve Safety

Here's what trauma might have taught you: safety is conditional. You have to earn it. You have to be good enough, healed enough, together enough.

Here's the truth: Safety is your birthright. You deserved it as a child and didn't get it. You deserve it now and can create it. Not perfect safety—that doesn't exist. But enough safety to breathe, to heal, to build a life that feels worth living.

Start where you are. Use what you have. Do what you can. Every small act of self-protection is a victory. Every boundary you set is healing. Every time you choose safety over familiarity, you're rewriting your story.

You don't need to be further along in healing to deserve safety. You deserve it now. You matter now. And every step toward safety is a step toward freedom.

Coaching Corner: Safety as Sacred Ground

Think of safety like tending a garden. You can't make flowers bloom by force, but you can create the conditions where growth becomes possible. Every safety measure you put in place—every boundary, every grounding tool, every supportive relationship—is like preparing the soil. You're not just protecting yourself from harm; you're creating sacred ground where your healing can take root and flourish.

Some days you'll be planting, some days watering, some days just protecting what's already there from storms. All of it matters. All of it is sacred work. Your safety isn't selfish—it's the foundation everything else gets built on.

PART VII: DISCLOSURE AND SUPPORT

Sharing Your Story and Getting Help

27

Disclosure: When, Why, and How to Tell Your Story

Telling someone what happened doesn't make you weak. It means you're ready for the weight to be shared.

Y OU'VE CARRIED THIS SECRET like a stone in your chest. Maybe for months, maybe for decades. The weight of it affects every breath, every relationship, every quiet moment. And now you're here, holding the possibility of telling someone. That's huge. It means your need for healing is beginning to outweigh your fear.

But the questions swirl: "Do I have to tell someone to heal?" "What if they don't believe me?" "What if everything changes?" "What if I regret it?" "What if it makes things worse?"

This chapter isn't about pushing you to disclose before you're ready. There's no timetable, no requirement, no "should." This is about understanding what disclosure means, how to do it as safely as possible, and how to reclaim your voice—on your terms, at your pace.

What Disclosure Really Means

Disclosure is simply telling someone about your abuse. It can take countless forms: a whispered confession to a friend, a letter you hand to someone silently, three words: "It happened to me," a text that says "I need to tell you something," details shared with a therapist, your story told in a support group, writing "me too" on social media, or a journal entry you read aloud.

Disclosure can be private (told to one trusted person), selective (shared with a few safe people), public (shared openly through social media or advocacy), partial ("something happened" without details), or complete (the full story with names and specifics).

There's no hierarchy here. Telling one person "something bad happened" is just as valid as telling your whole story publicly. Your disclosure belongs to you.

Why Telling Can Help (And Why It's Not Required)

Let's be clear: you can absolutely heal without telling anyone. Many survivors do. Healing is internal work that doesn't require external validation. But many survivors also find that disclosure becomes a turning point because it breaks the silence. Secrets have power, and speaking truth, even to one person, can feel like setting down a weight you've carried too long.

It interrupts shame. Shame thrives in darkness. When you speak your truth and someone responds with care, shame begins to lose its grip.

It creates connection. Carrying trauma alone is exhausting. Letting someone share even a tiny piece can feel like oxygen.

It validates your experience. Sometimes we need to hear our own story out loud to believe it really happened, that it really mattered.

It opens doors to support. People can't help with what they don't know about. Disclosure can connect you to resources and care.

But remember: these benefits only come when disclosure is YOUR choice, on YOUR timeline, to people YOU trust.

Why Disclosure Feels Impossible

Most survivors take years—sometimes decades—to tell anyone. The reasons are completely valid.

Fear of not being believed: "What if they think I'm lying or exaggerating?" **Fear of being blamed:** "What if they ask what I was wearing or why I didn't fight back?" **Fear of losing relationships:** "What if they choose my abuser over me?" **Fear of the consequences:** "What if this tears my family apart?" **Fear of losing control:** "What if they tell everyone or make me report it?" **Fear of feeling it again:** "What if saying it out loud makes it real again?"

These fears aren't irrational. Many survivors have experienced these exact outcomes. That's why preparing carefully matters.

> **Somatic Exercise for Pre-Disclosure Grounding:** Before any disclosure conversation, try this: Stand with your back against a wall. Press your whole spine against it, feeling the solid support. Take three deep breaths. Step away from the wall but imagine that support is still with you—like wearing an invisible shield of protection. This helps your body remember you have backing, even in vulnerable moments.

Testing the Waters

You don't have to start with full disclosure. You can test how safe someone might be:

Use hypothetical questions: "What would you do if a friend told you something really hard?" "Do you think victims of abuse should always report?" "How do you think families should handle it when abuse happens?"

Try sharing adjacent stories: "I read this article about trauma..." "I have a friend who went through something..." "I've been thinking a lot about how common abuse is..."

Consider partial disclosure: "I've been dealing with something from my past," "Something happened when I was younger that still affects me," or "I experienced some trauma I'm working through."

Watch how they respond. Do they listen? Do they blame victims? Do they change the subject? Their responses tell you whether they're safe for deeper disclosure.

Choosing Who to Tell

Start with the safest person possible. Look for someone who has shown empathy in other situations. Choose someone who listens more than they talk. Find someone who doesn't try to fix everything. Look for someone who respects boundaries. Choose someone who keeps confidences. Pick someone who believes in you.

This might be a therapist or counselor, a trusted friend, a teacher or mentor, a support group, a crisis hotline (this can be anonymous), or an online survivor community.

How to Tell: Scripts and Strategies

Having words ready can help when emotions run high:

Opening the conversation: "I have something difficult I need to share," "This is hard to say, but I trust you," "I've never told anyone this before," or "Can I tell you something without you trying to fix it?"

The disclosure itself: "When I was [age], someone hurt me sexually," "I was abused by [relationship without name if it feels safer]," "Something happened that I'm still processing," or "I experienced sexual trauma."

Setting boundaries: "I'm not ready to share details," "Please don't ask questions right now," "I need you to keep this between us," or "I just need you to listen, not advise."

If writing feels safer: Sometimes writing lets you say what your voice can't. You can write a letter and hand it to them in person. You can send a text message or email when you're ready. You can write your thoughts while you're together and show them. Or you can prepare notes ahead of time and read from them during the conversation.

Preparing for Different Responses

Best case responses: "I believe you," "This wasn't your fault," "Thank you for trusting me," "How can I support you?" or "I'm here for whatever you need."

Challenging responses: They might show shock or silence because they need time to process. They might ask too many questions, but you can set boundaries. They might try to "fix" things immediately, so redirect them to just listening. They might make it about themselves, so gently refocus the conversation.

Harmful responses: Some people won't believe you. Others will minimize what happened. Some might blame you. Others will make you feel ashamed. Some will pressure you to report it. Others will push you to confront your abuser. Some might break your confidentiality. They could tell people without permission. Some will make excuses for the person who hurt you.

If someone responds harmfully, remember—their response reflects who they are, not the truth of what happened to you. When someone dismisses your experience, blames you, or refuses to believe you, they're showing you their own limitations, fears, and inability to handle difficult truths. Their reaction says everything about their character, their capacity for empathy, and their willingness to sit with uncomfortable realities. It says nothing about whether your experience was real, whether you deserved what happened, or whether you're worthy of support. A harmful response is never about you—it's always about them.

After You Tell

Disclosure can bring relief, but it can also bring vulnerability hangover. Plan for aftercare:

Immediate after-care: Have a comfort plan (bath, walk, favorite show). Don't make big decisions right away. Be gentle with yourself. Remember – you can't "take it back" but you can control what happens next.

Following days: You might feel exposed or regretful – this is normal. You might feel relief or lightness – this is normal too. Check in with your body and emotions. Reach out to other support people if needed (trusted friends, family members, counselor, or support groups).

If You're Not Ready

Then don't. Full stop. You don't owe anyone your story. Healing can happen without disclosure. You can write it in a journal just for you, tell your story to an empty room, share anonymously online, work through it in therapy without naming names, or create art that expresses without words.

Your timeline is the right timeline.

Special Considerations

Family disclosure is often the most complex. This is especially true if the abuser is family. It's complicated when they're still in contact with the abuser. It's harder when they have their own trauma. Family reputation might matter more to them than your truth. You don't owe family automatic disclosure. Your safety comes first.

Partner disclosure doesn't have to happen immediately. You don't have to disclose to romantic partners right away. You can share general information like "I have some trauma history." You can explain behavioral needs like "I need to go slow physically." You can set boundaries without giving explanations.

Professional disclosure gives you control over details. When telling teachers, doctors, or other professionals, you choose how much to share. Focus on what you need from them. Remember confidentiality limits like mandated reporting requirements.

Mandated reporting means certain professionals are legally required to report suspected abuse to authorities. This includes teachers, doctors, nurses, therapists, social workers, and childcare providers. They must report if they believe a child is currently being abused or if an adult discloses abuse of a child. However, if you're an adult disclosing your own childhood abuse that happened in the past and no children are currently at risk, this typically doesn't trigger mandatory reporting. Laws vary by state, so it's okay to ask professionals about their reporting requirements before you share details. You can also focus your disclosure on current symptoms and what support you need rather than specific abuse details.

The Power of Your Voice

Whether you whisper your truth to one person or shout it from rooftops, your story is yours. Whether you tell today or in twenty years or never, it belongs to you. No one can take that from you.

Disclosure isn't about owing anyone your pain. It's about choosing when to share the burden you've been carrying. It's about choosing how to share it. It's about choosing if you want to share it at all. It's about discovering that your voice still works. Your voice was silenced for so long. But it still matters.

A Gentle Reminder

You are not required to tell anyone for your story or feelings to be valid. Your healing doesn't depend on others knowing. Your worth isn't determined by who believes you.

But you are also allowed to want to be known. To crave the relief of sharing. To need the connection that comes from being seen in your truth.

Whatever you choose—silence or speech, privacy or publicity, partial truths or full disclosure—let it be YOUR choice. Let it serve YOUR healing. Let it honor YOUR journey.

Your story is sacred. Handle it with the care it deserves. Share it with those who've earned the privilege. And remember: speaking your truth is not betrayal—it's freedom.

Whether you tell today, tomorrow, or never... your story is real. You are not broken. And you are allowed to move toward freedom—at your own pace, in your own way.

You do not owe your pain to anyone. But you are allowed to release it.

Coaching Corner: Your Story, Your Power

Your story has been held hostage by silence, but here's the truth: you hold all the keys. Every time you choose who to tell, what to share, when to speak—you're exercising power that trauma tried to steal. Disclosure isn't about giving your story away; it's about choosing to let others witness it.

Like a precious artifact in a museum, you decide who gets close enough to see, who can be trusted with its beauty and its pain. Some will earn the privilege of the full exhibit. Others might only see one piece through protective glass. And some will never be allowed in at all. That's not secrecy—that's sovereignty. Your story, your rules, your power.

28

When Abuse Happens by Christians: Facing Spiritual Betrayal

When someone uses God's name to hurt you, they wound not just your body, but your very soul.

ABUSE WOUNDS DEEPLY NO matter who commits it. But when your abuser claimed to represent God—when they prayed with you, quoted Scripture to you, held spiritual authority over you—the wound cuts into your very soul. It's not just personal betrayal. It's cosmic betrayal.

If you were harmed by someone who called themselves a Christian, especially a leader or someone your faith community trusted, you're likely carrying questions that feel too dangerous to ask:

Where was God when it happened? Did God allow this? Can I ever trust spiritual authority again? Am I still allowed to be angry? Is my faith ruined forever?

This chapter is for those navigating the unique devastation of spiritual abuse intertwined with sexual abuse. You're not alone in this struggle, and your questions aren't blasphemous—they're necessary.

Understanding Spiritual Abuse

Spiritual abuse happens when someone uses God, faith, Scripture, or religious authority to manipulate, control, or harm others. When sexual abuse comes wrapped in spiritual language, it creates layers of confusion that can take years to untangle.

This might look like using Scripture to justify abuse ("Wives submit," "Honor your father," "Forgive seventy times seven"), claiming the abuse is "God's will" or part of His plan, saying God told them to do it, using spiritual language to groom ("You're special to God," "This is holy"), threatening spiritual consequences ("You'll go to hell if you tell"), weaponizing forgiveness to silence victims, or using their position to access and abuse.

Dr. Dan Allender puts it powerfully: "All sexual abuse is spiritual abuse, even when God's name is never mentioned." Why? Because abuse always attacks the *imago Dei*—the image of God within you. It assaults your inherent dignity and worth.

Why Spiritual Abuse Devastates Differently

When abuse comes from someone representing God, the damage goes beyond the personal:

It distorts God's character. The abuser becomes the lens through which you see God. If they were controlling, God feels controlling. If they were cruel, God feels cruel. If they abandoned you, God feels absent.

It weaponizes sacred things. Scripture, prayer, worship, communion—things meant to bring life become triggers. Church feels dangerous. The Bible feels like a weapon. Prayer feels impossible.

It isolates you from spiritual community. Where do you go when your faith community IS the unsafe place? Who do you tell when the abuser is revered by everyone? How do you report "God's anointed"?

It attacks your core identity. If you found identity in being a "child of God," and someone representing God violated you, who are you now? The very foundation of self gets shaken.

It creates theological confusion. You might wrestle with questions like: "Did I sin by 'participating'?" "Is God punishing me?" "Have I lost my salvation?" "Am I too defiled for God now?"

God's Actual View on Abuse

Let's be crystal clear about what Scripture actually says:

God is furious about abuse. Throughout the Bible, God consistently defends the vulnerable (Psalm 82:3), rages against those who harm others (Matthew 18:6), stands with the oppressed (Isaiah 1:17), grieves with the brokenhearted (Psalm 34:18), and promises justice for abusers (Romans 12:19).

Jesus himself protected children fiercely, elevated women's dignity, confronted religious abuse and corruption, sided with victims over reputation, and experienced abuse and betrayal personally. When Jesus found people being exploited and taken advantage of in the temple, he didn't stay quiet to keep the peace—he overturned tables and drove out those who were harming others.

The God revealed in Jesus is nothing like your abuser. Your abuser lied about who God is. They used God's name in vain in the deepest way possible.

Common Lies Told by "Christian" Abusers

Recognizing these lies can help you separate your abuser's voice from God's truth:

"This is how God shows love" **Truth:** God's love never violates, never forces, never shames.

"You must forgive and forget immediately" **Truth:** Forgiveness is a journey, not a demanded instant response. And forgiveness never requires reconciliation with an unsafe person.

"If you tell, you'll destroy God's work" **Truth:** Exposing abuse doesn't destroy God's work—abuse does. Truth brings healing.

"Your body made me stumble" **Truth:** Your body is not responsible for someone else's sin. Ever.

"God won't love you if you're not pure" **Truth:** Nothing can separate you from God's love. Nothing.

"Submit to authority no matter what" **Truth:** God never calls you to submit to abuse. Biblical submission is mutual and protective, never harmful.

Reclaiming Faith After Spiritual Betrayal

Healing from spiritual abuse often means deconstructing false beliefs before reconstructing healthy faith:

Separate the abuser from God. They claimed to represent God but they lied. God looks like Jesus—compassionate, protective, just, gentle with the wounded.

Find safe spiritual spaces. Look for communities that prioritize survivor safety over reputation, have transparent accountability, don't rush forgiveness, understand trauma, and allow questions and anger.

Reclaim Scripture. You might need to take a break from triggering passages, read with trauma-informed resources, focus on God's justice and protection, and let yourself see God as defender, not attacker.

Express your anger. The Psalms are full of rage, questions, and accusations toward God. You're allowed to be honest about your pain. God can handle your anger—it's often the beginning of healing.

Consider trauma-informed spiritual direction. Some counselors specialize in religious trauma. They can help you separate authentic faith from spiritual abuse.

Consider writing a letter to God expressing your honest questions and anger. Write out the lies your abuser told you about faith, then beside each one, write what you now believe to be true. Sometimes we need to see the contrast on paper to separate twisted theology from authentic faith. See Chapter 14.

Red Flags in Faith Communities

As you heal, watch for these warning signs in religious spaces:

Leaders who can't be questioned

Emphasis on reputation over righteousness

Victim-blaming theology

Rushed forgiveness without justice

Secrecy and lack of accountability

Controlling behavior disguised as "discipleship"

Using Scripture to silence or shame

You deserve faith communities that feel safe, where questions are welcomed, where survivors are believed, where healing is prioritized over appearances.

What Healing Can Look Like

Embodied Spirituality: Religious trauma sometimes creates disconnection from the body, viewing it as "sinful" or "shameful." True spiritual healing includes honoring your body as sacred. The body awareness practices from Chapter 1 can help you reclaim your physical self as part of your spiritual journey.

Spiritual healing after religious abuse is possible, though the path is unique for each survivor:

For some: Complete break from organized religion while maintaining personal spirituality

For others: Finding new faith communities that feel safe

For many: Deconstructing harmful theology while reconstructing life-giving faith

For all: Learning that you are not defined by what happened, that your worth remains intact, that you are beloved exactly as you are

If You're Still in It

If you're currently in an abusive situation with spiritual elements:

Your safety matters more than their reputation

You can leave, even if they say God forbids it

You can report, even if they're a leader

You can get help, even if they've isolated you

God is not honored by your suffering

Resources for Healing

Consider these specialized resources:

The Wounded Heart by Dr. Dan Allender

Redeeming Power by Diane Langberg

Something's Not Right by Wade Mullen

The Allender Center for trauma and faith

Support groups for religious trauma

Therapists who understand spiritual abuse

A Final Word

Your abuser stole many things—innocence, safety, trust. But they couldn't steal your inherent worth. They couldn't steal God's actual love for you. They couldn't steal your right to heal.

You may feel like your faith is in ruins. Maybe it is. But sometimes things need to be demolished before they can be rebuilt properly. The faith you reconstruct—if you choose to—can be yours. Not theirs. Not the institution's. Yours.

Whether you find your way back to faith or find peace apart from it, know this: you are not damaged goods in God's eyes. You are not too broken for love. You are not defined by what someone did in God's name.

You are beloved. You are worthy. You are held.

Even in the ruins. Especially in the ruins.

That's where resurrection happens.

Coaching Corner: Sacred Reconstruction

When spiritual abuse happens, it's like someone taking a sledge-hammer to a cathedral. The destruction can feel complete, devastating, final. But here's what I want you to know: even in the rubble, the foundation remains. Your worth, your belovedness, your connection to the Divine—these aren't housed in buildings or held by people. They're built into your very being.

Sometimes reconstruction means building something entirely different on that foundation. Sometimes it means restoring what was beautiful before someone destroyed it. Sometimes it means leaving the space open to the sky for a while, letting healing happen in the elements. All of these are sacred. All of these honor what remains unbreakable in you.

29

Working with a Therapist or Coach: Finding the Right Fit for Your Healing

"Healing doesn't happen in isolation. It happens in connection." Judith Herman

I F YOU'RE READING THIS book, it's likely because you're navigating trauma largely on your own—or you've tried to get help and it didn't feel right. That's okay. Healing can start within you, and it's incredibly brave to take those first steps solo. But it's also true that having a guide—a therapist, coach, or mentor—can help you go further, faster, and safer.

This chapter will help you understand the difference between therapists and coaches, learn what kind of support might be best for you, spot red and green flags in professional helpers, prepare for your first sessions, and trust your instincts in the process.

You Deserve Safe Support

Working with a professional doesn't mean you're broken. It means you're wise enough to want support.

Healing from sexual trauma often involves uncovering and releasing memories, emotions, and patterns you didn't choose. It's okay if that feels overwhelming. Professionals trained in trauma can help you navigate those layers at your pace, with compassion and without judgment.

Therapist vs. Coach: What's the Difference?

Therapists are trained mental health professionals. They may be licensed counselors (LPC), psychologists (PhD or PsyD), clinical social workers (LCSW), or marriage and family therapists (LMFT). Therapists can diagnose and treat mental health conditions, are trained in trauma-specific methods (like EMDR, somatic experiencing, IFS), often work through insurance or private pay, and may take a clinical, long-term approach.

Coaches are not licensed mental health professionals but are trained to support mindset, motivation, and emotional growth. Trauma-informed coaches help clients shift thinking patterns and beliefs, focus on the present and future, offer tools, structure, and accountability, and may specialize in areas like life direction, body image, identity, or empowerment.

What Kind of Help Do I Need?

Here's a quick tool to check what kind of support might best fit your current season:

"I have panic attacks or flashbacks I can't control." **Therapist**

"I want to stop self-harming or using substances to cope." **Therapist**

"I've never told anyone and don't know where to begin." **Therapist** or **trauma-informed coach**

"I want to reclaim my identity, confidence, and future." **Trauma-informed coach**

"I'm struggling with suicidal thoughts." **Therapist** or crisis support immediately

"I need tools to manage anxiety, boundaries, or self-worth." **Either therapist** or **trauma-informed coach**

Red Flags in Helping Professionals

They blame you for the abuse, rush you to talk about trauma before you feel ready, minimize your feelings, seem uncomfortable discussing sexual trauma, act distracted, judgmental, or impatient, push their own beliefs or agenda onto you, or don't explain their methods or respect your pace.

Green Flags: What Safe Support Looks Like

They validate your story and your feelings, honor your pace and ask for your consent, help you feel calm and grounded, offer structure, tools, and education, are open about their training and methods, welcome your feedback, and make you feel seen, not "fixed."

What to Ask Before You Begin

"Have you worked with survivors of sexual trauma?" "What trauma-informed methods do you use?" "How do you create a sense of safety in your sessions?" "Do you support clients who haven't disclosed their trauma to anyone else?" "How do you respond if someone dissociates or has a flashback during session?"

Preparing for the First Session

You don't have to tell everything at once. You can say: "I've been through something hard. I'm not ready to talk about it all, but I'd like help with how it's affecting me now," "I think I have trauma, but I don't have clear memories," or "This is my first time getting support, and I feel nervous."

If You Had a Bad Experience Before

If you've seen a therapist or coach before and it didn't help—or made things worse—you are not the problem.

Unfortunately, many survivors have stories of being dismissed, misunderstood, or even harmed by well-meaning (or not so well-meaning) professionals.

It's okay to try again. It doesn't have to be the same this time.

What Healing Together Looks Like

Support doesn't mean giving away your power—it means learning how to hold it again.

Whether you work with a licensed trauma therapist, a somatic practitioner, a Christian life coach, or a trusted guide—healing can deepen when it's shared. You're not weak for needing support. You're wise.

You don't have to do this alone.

Optional Reflection: Journal Prompt: What kind of support feels safest to you right now—clinical, creative, spiritual, relational, or educational? What would your ideal helper say to you on your hardest day?

Coaching Corner: Your Healing Team

Think of building your support team like assembling a crew for an important expedition. You wouldn't climb Everest alone, and you don't have to navigate trauma recovery solo either. Some team members might be there for the whole journey—the base camp managers who know your story and hold steady presence. Others might join for specific sections—the technical climbers who help you navigate particularly challenging terrain.

Your healing team might include a therapist, a coach, (I'm honored when survivors choose to include me in their healing journey) a trusted friend, a support group, a spiritual director, or a bodyworker. There's no "right" combination, only what serves your unique path. The key is choosing people who believe in your capacity to heal and who walk alongside you without trying to carry you or push you up the mountain faster than you're ready to climb.

30

Early Abuse, Same-Sex Attraction, and Gender Identity

Your identity is yours to discover, define, and embrace— regardless of what influenced its development.

THIS CHAPTER IS WRITTEN with deep care and respect for every reader, regardless of where you are in understanding your sexuality or gender identity. It's a complex topic that deserves nuance, compassion, and the acknowledgment that your journey is yours alone.

Many survivors carry silent questions about whether their sexual orientation or gender identity might be connected to early abuse. If you've wondered about this, you're not alone. These questions don't make you broken, confused, or wrong. They make you human, trying to understand yourself in the aftermath of trauma.

This chapter isn't about telling you who you are or why you are. It's about creating space to explore how trauma can complicate our understanding of ourselves, while honoring wherever that exploration leads you.

The Complexity We're Navigating

When sexual abuse happens during childhood or adolescence—those crucial years when we're developing our sense of self, our relationship to our bodies, and our understanding of intimacy—it can affect how these aspects of identity form. This doesn't mean abuse "causes" any particular orientation or identity. It means trauma can complicate an already complex process.

Some survivors experience confusion about attraction and fear, questions about whether their desires are "authentic" or trauma-based, disconnection from their bodies or assigned gender, uncertainty about what feelings are "normal," or fear that their identity is somehow "wrong" or "damaged."

These experiences deserve compassion, not judgment.

Same-Sex Attraction After Abuse

For some survivors, particularly those abused by someone of the same gender, questions about sexual orientation can feel especially loaded: "Did the abuse make me gay?" "Would I feel this way if it hadn't happened?" "How do I know what's real attraction versus trauma response?" "Am I drawn to the familiar, even if it was harmful?"

Let's be clear: sexual orientation isn't caused by abuse. Many people who were never abused identify as LGBTQ+. Many who were abused identify as straight. The relationship between trauma and identity is far more nuanced than simple cause and effect.

What we do know is that trauma can blur the lines between fear and arousal, create confusion about safety and attraction, lead to seeking the familiar even when harmful, and affect how we understand intimacy and connection.

This doesn't invalidate your feelings or attractions. It simply acknowledges that trauma can add layers of complexity to an already personal journey.

> **Somatic Exercise for Identity Exploration:** Sit comfortably and place both hands over your heart. Breathe deeply and ask yourself, "Who am I when I feel safest?" Don't force an answer. Just notice what arises—feelings, images, sensations. This isn't about finding "the answer" but about creating space for your authentic self to speak, free from trauma's noise.

Gender Identity and Body Relationship

Some survivors describe feeling disconnected from their assigned gender after abuse. This might manifest as rejecting aspects of femininity or masculinity that feel vulnerable, feeling safer presenting as a different gender, experiencing dysphoria that may or may not be related to trauma, wanting to be invisible or ungendered, or feeling like their body betrayed them.

For example, a survivor assigned female at birth might reject femininity because it was targeted. A survivor assigned male might disconnect from masculinity if it's associated with their abuser. Any survivor might feel safer in a body that seems less vulnerable to abuse.

These responses make sense as protective strategies. They don't necessarily define your core gender identity, but they're valid responses to trauma that deserve exploration, not dismissal.

The Challenge of Untangling

One of the hardest parts of this journey is trying to separate what might be trauma response, what might be authentic identity, and whether that separation even matters.

The truth is, you might never fully untangle these threads—and that's okay. Your identity is valid regardless of what influenced its development. We're all shaped by our experiences. Trauma survivors don't owe anyone a "pure" origin story for their identity.

Questions for Gentle Exploration

If you're navigating these questions, consider exploring:

About attraction: Do I feel drawn to people who feel safe or familiar? Can I distinguish between fear and attraction? What happens in my body when I feel attracted to someone? Do my attractions feel like choices or compulsions?

About gender: When do I feel most comfortable in my body? What aspects of gender feel authentic versus protective? How did I understand my gender before the abuse? What would feeling safe in my body look like?

About identity overall: Am I exploring from a place of curiosity or survival? What identities feel expansive versus restrictive? Who am I when I feel safest? What would I choose if I weren't afraid?

These aren't questions with right or wrong answers. They're invitations to know yourself more deeply.

For Those Raised in Religious Contexts

If you were raised in a faith tradition with specific teachings about sexuality and gender, you might carry additional layers: fear that questioning means failing spiritually, belief that certain identities are inherently wrong, confusion about whether God still loves you, pressure to "choose" heterosexuality or traditional gender expression, or shame about normal exploration and questioning.

Remember: questioning doesn't make you faithless. God is not threatened by your honest questions or confusion. He understands that trauma can cloud our understanding of ourselves and create genuine uncertainty about who we are.

As you navigate these questions, consider that God created you with intention and love. While trauma may have confused your understanding of yourself, it didn't change how God made you. This doesn't mean questioning is wrong - it means your questions can become prayers, and your confusion can become an invitation to seek God's voice about who He says you are.

Some find it helpful to bring their questions directly to God in prayer, seek counsel from mature believers who understand both trauma and faith. Remember that God's love for you isn't dependent on having everything figured out, and trust that seeking truth about your identity can be an act of worship.

Each person's journey through these questions looks different. Some find clarity quickly; others wrestle longer. What matters is remaining open to God's voice about who He created you to be, even when trauma has made that voice harder to hear. Your worth isn't determined by having immediate answers, but neither are you meant to walk this path without divine guidance.

The Path Forward

Healing doesn't mean arriving at a fixed identity that never questions or shifts. It means developing a compassionate relationship with yourself, creating safety to explore without judgment, distinguishing between survival responses and authentic desires, accepting that some questions might not have clear answers, and choosing identities that help you thrive, not just survive.

Whether you ultimately identify as LGBTQ+ and see that as unrelated to trauma, LGBTQ+ and recognize trauma's influence without invalidating your identity, straight and working through trauma-based confusion, or fluid, questioning, or resistant to labels entirely—your journey is valid. Your identity is yours to define.

Working with Professionals

If you choose to explore these questions with professional support, look for therapists who are both trauma-informed AND LGBTQ+-affirming, professionals who don't push any particular outcome, provided space to explore without judgment or agenda, understand that identity can be fluid and complex, and display respect for your self-determination.

Avoid anyone who claims abuse "causes" homosexuality, promises to "fix" your orientation or gender identity, dismisses either trauma's impact OR identity validity, or makes you feel shame about questions or exploration.

Integration and Acceptance

Ultimately, healing might not mean finding definitive answers to all your questions. It might mean accepting the complexity of your experience, choosing identities that help you feel whole, building relationships that honor all parts of you, creating safety in your body regardless of labels, and trusting yourself to know what feels authentic.

You don't owe anyone—including yourself—a simple story. Your identity is allowed to be complex, influenced by many factors, and still completely valid.

A Final Thought

Whether trauma influenced your identity or not, whether you're certain about who you are or still exploring—you deserve love, acceptance, and the space to be fully yourself. Your questions don't make you broken. Your exploration doesn't make you confused. Your identity—however you understand it—doesn't need to be defended or justified.

You are whole, worthy, and welcome in this world exactly as you are. Your journey to understand yourself is sacred, and you get to walk it at your own pace, in your own way.

There's no timeline for figuring yourself out. There's no requirement to have clear answers. There's only your life, your truth, and your right to live it authentically—whatever that means for you.

You are enough, exactly as you are, in all your complexity.

Coaching Corner: The Journey Is the Destination

We live in a world that demands labels, clear answers, definitive identities. But here's a secret: the questioning itself is sacred. The exploration is the point. Whether you're wondering about orientation, gender, or any aspect of identity, the courage to ask "Who am I?" is more important than any answer you might find.

Some survivors spend years trying to separate what's "trauma" from what's "real," as if they're opposing forces. But what if they're both real? What if you're allowed to be a complex human whose identity is influenced by many things—including but not limited to trauma? Your identity doesn't need to be pure to be valid. It just needs to be yours. And the beautiful thing about it being yours? You get to keep exploring, changing, growing, and becoming for as long as you live. That's not confusion. That's freedom.

Conclusion: Your Path Forward

Hey. You made it to the end. That's huge.

MAYBE YOU READ EVERY word, or maybe you jumped around to the parts that felt safest. Maybe some chapters made you want to throw this book across the room. Maybe you cried, or felt numb, or had to take breaks. However you got here—it counts. It all counts.

I'm sitting here writing this last chapter, thinking about all the survivors who will read these words—those drowning in shame and secrets, whose bodies feel like enemies they're stuck living with, who are convinced they'll never feel normal or happy or whole again.

If that's you, I want you to know what I wish every survivor could hear in their darkest moments: where you are right now isn't where you'll always be. I know that might sound like empty words, especially if you're in the thick of it. But I promise you—it's true.

Where We've Been Together

We've covered a lot in these pages. You've learned how trauma actually works and why you're not "crazy" for feeling the way you do. You've learned ways to calm your body when it goes into panic mode. You've discovered the truth that you're worthy even when your brain lies and says you're not. You've learned how to catch those nasty thoughts and flip them. You know what to do when memories crash into your day. You understand why the shame you're carrying was never yours to hold. You've seen how writing can help when talking feels impossible. You've found ways to discover joy and creativity again. You've learned the power of saying "no" and meaning it. You know that safe people exist even if you haven't found them yet. And you've learned that you still get to have dreams and a future.

Your body's been through a lot. It's been holding all this stuff—the fear, the memories, the need to stay on guard. But here's the thing: your body's not broken. It's been doing its best to protect you with the tools it had. Now you're giving it new tools, better tools. You're teaching it that it's okay to relax sometimes. That not everyone is dangerous. That you deserve to take up space in the world.

Let Me Tell You About Noah

Maybe parts of Noah's story are yours too.

When Noah was 11, his parents' friend—this guy everyone thought was so great—took him camping. The summer air hung thick with humidity, and the tent fabric stuck to his skin as he tried to sleep. What happened in that cramped space, with the distant sound of crickets chirping and the musty smell of canvas surrounding them, changed everything. The man made Noah promise to keep their "special game" secret, said Noah's parents would hate him if they knew. The weight of those words pressed down on Noah's chest like a stone he'd carry for years. So Noah locked it all inside.

Fast forward to 16. Noah felt like a ghost walking through his own life. The fluorescent lights in school hallways seemed too bright, voices sounded muffled like he was underwater, and his own reflection in bathroom mirrors looked foreign. He'd lose it over tiny things—a dropped pencil, a slammed locker—then hate himself for being "too sensitive." He couldn't concentrate. His body felt heavy and wrong, like he was wearing a costume that didn't fit. Sometimes he'd scratch his arms raw just to feel something real, something that proved he was still there.

One random Tuesday, Noah was hiding in the library (safer than the cafeteria, where laughter felt like mockery and the smell of pizza made his stomach turn) when he found this book about trauma and healing. His hands shook as he flipped through it, the pages whispering secrets he'd never heard spoken aloud. Some parts made him want to run. But other parts... it was like reading his own thoughts for the first time.

He started small. Really small. One breathing exercise when the bathroom walls felt like they were closing in. Three words in a notebook at night: "I survived today." The ink looked bold against the white page, proof of something he couldn't quite name yet. That's it.

Week by week, Noah started noticing things. How his jaw clenched during certain conversations. How his breath got shallow when he passed that camping gear store downtown, the smell of canvas and rope triggering something deep in his chest. He wasn't "fixing" himself—he was just paying attention.

Photography club was a random choice, but holding a camera felt good. The weight of it in his hands was grounding, solid. He got to decide what to focus on, what to leave out of frame. Control, but the good kind. His friend Jamie noticed he'd been quiet lately and said, "Hey, if you ever need to talk... or not talk but just hang out... I'm around." Noah wasn't ready to spill everything, but knowing someone saw him—really saw him—without pushing? That was everything.

Now Noah's saving money for a real camera. He dreams about traveling, capturing moments of beauty—sunrise over mountains, children laughing in parks, the way light filters through autumn leaves. The future used to feel like something to survive. Now it feels like something to build.

Your story might be different. Your pain might look different. But the path forward? It's made of the same small, brave steps.

What You're Taking With You

Everything in this book is yours now. Not homework you have to perfect, just tools you can grab when you need them.

Recognizing trauma helps you stop wondering "what's wrong with me?" and start understanding "this is how my body learned to protect itself." Breathing exercises become your emergency brake when everything speeds up. Self-worth reminders are there for when shame gets loud. Thought flips matter because the mean voice in your head lies a lot. Grounding techniques ensure flashbacks don't win. Shame-busting reminds you that shame belongs to who hurt you, not you. Writing is cheaper than therapy and always available. Creative activities prove your body can still make good things. Boundaries mean your space, your rules. Connection matters because isolation makes everything worse. Hope remains the most rebellious thing you can choose.

Look, I know sometimes it all feels too big. Maybe you've hurt yourself trying to make the inside pain stop. Maybe you've cut, or burned, or found other ways to feel something else—anything else—for just a minute. If that's you, you're not bad or weak or crazy. You were just trying to survive with the tools you had.

But those tools come with a cost, right? The relief never lasts long enough, and usually you end up feeling worse. So here's something else to try: pause three times today and just notice your body. Not judge it—just notice. Tight shoulders? Clenched stomach? Relaxed hands? Just notice. You're building a relationship with your body instead of a war against it.

When the urge to hurt yourself hits, try something else first. Hold ice cubes till they melt. Draw on your skin with a red marker. Do push-ups till your arms shake. Scream into a pillow. It won't feel the same at first. That's okay. You're learning a new language—the language of taking care of yourself instead of punishing yourself.

Why This Matters (Like, Really Matters)

Someone hurt you, and that sucks. It's unfair and wrong and it shouldn't have happened. And you did not deserve it! You are valuable beyond measure and loved more than words can describe. But here's what I know now that I didn't know then: the trauma doesn't have to be the end of your story. It can be a chapter—a hard, painful chapter—but not the whole book.

When you were little, you did what you had to do to get through it. Maybe you shut down. Maybe you fought. Maybe you froze. Maybe you learned to handle everything alone because adults weren't safe. Whatever you did, it worked—you're here, reading this. You survived.

But now you get to do more than survive. You get to build a life where your body feels like home. Where relationships add to your life instead of threatening it. Where the future is something you're creating, not just enduring.

The stats say one in three girls and one in five boys go through some kind of sexual abuse. But in my conversations with people, I believe that number is higher. In any room, at any party, in any class—you're not the only one carrying this weight. But I know it feels lonely. Like everyone else is normal and you're walking around with this huge thing that makes you different. Separate. Less than.

That's trauma lying to you again. You're not less than anyone. You're not damaged goods. You're a person who survived something terrible and is fighting to heal. That's not weak—that's warrior-level strong.

What I Know Now

When I was young, I was sure the shame would suffocate me. I kept my mouth shut to protect everyone else's feelings, everyone else's comfort. Meanwhile, I was drowning in silence.

My healing journey didn't start until I was much older. For years, I carried that weight alone, thinking it was just how life would always be. My body held all that tension. I struggled in ways I couldn't even name back then.

What ultimately brought me healing was deeper than any single tool—it was finding forgiveness and discovering I was loved beyond measure. While that spiritual journey isn't the focus of this book, I want you to know that true, lasting healing is possible. The tools in these pages—breathing exercises, writing, body work—they're powerful support for you along the way. They can ease your pain, calm your panic, and help you reclaim your life.

I share these tools because I've seen them work. They help you manage the day-to-day, find your voice, and build strength. And maybe, as you use them, you'll find your own path to the deeper healing that transforms everything. Whether that comes through faith, therapy, community, or some combination—trust that it's out there waiting for you.

I help other people find their way through this darkness because I see so much unnecessary pain. I see so much hidden strength waiting to be discovered. And because I want you to know: you can build something beautiful from here. Your story isn't over. It's just beginning to turn toward hope.

The Last Thing (Promise)

You didn't deserve what happened to you. It wasn't your fault. Not even a little bit. Not even if you think you could have fought harder or screamed louder or done something different. It. Was. Not. Your. Fault.

The shame isn't yours. The blame isn't yours. The only thing that's yours is your future, and you get to decide what to do with it.

You don't have to forgive anyone. You don't have to be grateful for the "lessons." You don't have to find meaning in your pain. You just have to keep going, one breath at a time, one day at a time, one tiny victory at a time.

If you're ready for more support, it exists. That hotline I mentioned (1-800-656-HOPE or text RAINN to 741741) has people who get it. But if you're not ready, that's okay too. You've got tools now. You've got this book. You've got yourself, and that's not nothing.

You know what you deserve? To laugh without feeling guilty. To feel safe in your body. To trust people who earn it. To dream about your future and actually feel excited. To look in the mirror and not hate what you see. To be touched with kindness and not flinch. To take up space. To be loud. To be quiet. To be exactly who you are without apology.

That's not asking too much. That's asking for exactly what every human deserves. Including you. Especially you.

So keep going. Keep breathing. Keep trying these tools, even when they feel pointless. Keep choosing yourself, even in tiny ways. Because every time you do, you're proving that what happened to you doesn't get to write your ending.

You're writing it yourself. And I can't wait to see what you create.

You've got this. I promise.

About the Author

Agenna is first and foremost a follower of Christ, devoted wife of 35 years, and proud mother of three remarkable daughters. These foundations shape everything else she does—from her work as a Life and Mindset Coach at Coach Agenna to co-founding Brockley Co., a small business solutions company.

After her own journey through trauma recovery, Agenna discovered that true healing happens through honest acknowledgment of pain coupled with practical tools for moving forward. This revelation, combined with her faith, shaped her coaching philosophy: meet people where they are, believe their truth, and equip them with real strategies for real life.

She serves clients across all demographics and life stages—from executives and athletes to couples, survivors, students, and anyone seeking to break through barriers and build a stronger future. Whether helping an executive overcome limiting beliefs or a survivor reclaim their voice, she believes her clients are the experts of their own lives. Her role is to provide tools, support, and unwavering belief in their capacity to grow.

Through years of coaching, Agenna has witnessed incredible resilience across all areas of life. She's seen clients move from surviving to thriving—in boardrooms, on playing fields, in relationships, and in personal healing journeys. These transformations fuel her commitment to making powerful resources accessible to all who seek growth.

Beyond her professional work, Agenna serves her community by leading small groups focused on authentic connection and growth. As an active Toastmaster, she believes in the power of finding and using your voice. When time allows, she enjoys playing tennis and keeping up with the family's two energetic boxers.

Agenna attends Browns Bridge Church and lives with her family in North Georgia, where she remains inspired daily by God's grace and the courage of all those she's privileged to serve.

Connect with Agenna:

Website: agennamathley.com | healingwhathidesintheshadows.com

Email: agenna@agennamathley.com

Phone: 1-877-7agenna | 1(877)724-3662

"You are valuable beyond measure and loved more than words can describe. That's not just something I believe—it's something I know. And I wrote this book to help you know it too." Agenna

Author's Note Bibliography

Author's Note

THIS BOOK EXISTS BECAUSE of the groundbreaking work of trauma researchers who dared to challenge conventional wisdom and listen to what survivors' bodies were trying to tell us.

Dr. Bessel van der Kolk's research fundamentally changed how we understand trauma. His book "The Body Keeps the Score" provided the scientific foundation that validates what many survivors instinctively know—that trauma lives in the body, not just the mind. His emphasis on body-based healing, the importance of safety in recovery, and the understanding that we cannot heal while stuck in survival mode permeates every chapter of this book. Dr. van der Kolk's courage in challenging talk-therapy-only approaches opened the door for survivors to reclaim their bodies and their lives.

Dr. Peter Levine's work on Somatic Experiencing taught us that trauma is not a life sentence. His understanding of how the nervous system gets stuck and how it can be gently guided back to regulation forms the foundation of many exercises throughout this book. His insight that we can complete interrupted survival responses and help the body discharge trapped trauma energy has been revolutionary for countless survivors.

Dr. Gabor Maté's compassionate exploration of how trauma shapes us—not just psychologically but physically—has deepened our understanding of the mind-body connection. His work on how early experiences affect our stress response systems and his emphasis on self-compassion in healing have profoundly influenced the approach taken in this book.

This work also draws particularly on the pioneering somatic trauma research of Peter A. Levine and the parts-based trauma therapy approach of Janina Fisher, whose research on internal self-alienation and fragmented selves has significantly influenced the therapeutic framework presented here.

While I have adapted their insights specifically for survivors of sexual abuse and written from my own experience and understanding, the core wisdom belongs to these pioneering researchers. This book stands on the shoulders of their decades of research, clinical work, and advocacy for trauma survivors. Both works directly cited in the text and additional resources that informed the development of this book were selected for their contribution to trauma-informed healing and their accessibility to survivors seeking private recovery tools.

I encourage you to explore their work directly:

The Body Keeps the Score by Bessel van der Kolk MD —Essential reading for understanding how trauma affects the brain and body

Waking the Tiger by Peter Levine—A foundational text on how the body can heal from trauma

When the Body Says No by Gabor Maté—Explores the connection between stress, trauma, and physical illness

The Myth of Normal by Gabor Maté —A deeper dive into how trauma shapes our culture and individual lives

These books offer scientific depth and additional healing modalities that complement the practical tools in this book. Each researcher brings unique insights that can deepen your understanding of your own healing journey.

To every survivor reading this: your body is not broken. Your responses make sense. And healing is possible. These researchers proved it, and you can live it.

Here's your updated bibliography with the additional sources properly integrated:

Here's your updated bibliography with the additional sources properly integrated:

Bibliography & Reference List

Books Briere, J., & Scott, C. (2015). *Principles of Trauma Therapy: A Guide to Symptoms, Evaluation, and Treatment* (2nd ed.). Sage Publications.

Fisher, J. (2017). *Healing the Fragmented Selves of Trauma Survivors: Overcoming Internal Self-Alienation*. Routledge.

Herman, J. L. (1992). *Trauma and Recovery: The Aftermath of Violence—From Domestic Abuse to Political Terror*. Basic Books.

Levine, P. A. (1997). *Waking the Tiger: Healing Trauma—The Innate Capacity to Transform Overwhelming Experiences.* North Atlantic Books.

Levine, P. A. (2010). *In an Unspoken Voice: How the Body Releases Trauma and Restores Goodness.* North Atlantic Books.

Perry, B. D., & Winfrey, O. (2021). *What Happened to You? Conversations on Trauma, Resilience, and Healing.* Flatiron Books.

van der Kolk, B. A. (2014). *The Body Keeps the Score: Brain, Mind, and Body in the Healing of Trauma.* Viking.

Additional Resources Referenced Allender, D. B. (2008). *The Wounded Heart: Hope for Adult Victims of Childhood Sexual Abuse* (Rev. ed.). NavPress.

Bass, E., & Davis, L. (2008). *The Courage to Heal: A Guide for Women Survivors of Child Sexual Abuse* (4th ed.). Harper Paperbacks.

Brown, B. (2015). *Rising Strong: How the Ability to Reset Transforms the Way We Live, Love, Parent, and Lead.* Random House.

Fisher, J. (2021). *Transforming the Living Legacy of Trauma: A Workbook for Survivors and Therapists.* PESI Publishing.

Langberg, D. (2015). *Suffering and the Heart of God: How Trauma Destroys and Christ Restores.* New Growth Press.

Langberg, D. (2020). *Redeeming Power: Understanding Authority and Abuse in the Church.* Brazos Press.

Lew, M. (2004). *Victims No Longer: The Classic Guide for Men Recovering from Sexual Child Abuse* (2nd ed.). Harper Paperbacks.

Maltz, W. (2012). *The Sexual Healing Journey: A Guide for Survivors of Sexual Abuse* (3rd ed.). William Morrow Paperbacks.

Mullen, W. (2020). *Something's Not Right: Decoding the Hidden Tactics of Abuse and Freeing Yourself from Its Power.* Tyndale Momentum.

Walker, P. (2013). *Complex PTSD: From Surviving to Thriving.* Azure Coyote.

Book Chapters & Academic Sources Caffaro, J. V. (2014). *Sibling Abuse Trauma: Assessment and Intervention Strategies for Children, Families, and Adults.* Routledge.

Dube, S. R., Anda, R. F., Whitfield, C. L., Brown, D. W., Felitti, V. J., Dong, M., & Giles, W. H. (2005). Long-term consequences of childhood sexual abuse by gender of victim. *American Journal of Preventive Medicine,* 28(5), 430-438.

Felitti, V. J., Anda, R. F., Nordenberg, D., Williamson, D. F., Spitz, A. M., Edwards, V., Koss, M. P., & Marks, J. S. (1998). Relationship of childhood abuse and household dysfunction to many of the leading causes of death in adults: The Adverse Childhood Experiences (ACE) Study. *American Journal of Preventive Medicine,* 14(4), 245-258.

Finkelhor, D., Shattuck, A., Turner, H. A., & Hamby, S. L. (2014). The lifetime prevalence of child sexual abuse and sexual assault assessed in late adolescence. *Journal of Adolescent Health,* 55(3), 329-333. https://doi.org/10.1016/j.jadohealth.2014.02.006

Smith, S. G., Basile, K. C., Gilbert, L. K., Merrick, M. T., Patel, N., Walling, M., & Jain, A. (2017). *The National Intimate Partner and Sexual Violence*

Survey (NISVS): 2010-2012 State Report. National Center for Injury Prevention and Control, Centers for Disease Control and Prevention.

Online Resources Centers for Disease Control and Prevention. (2022). Adverse Childhood Experiences (ACEs). Retrieved January 15, 2025, from https://www.cdc.gov/violenceprevention/aces/index.html

RAINN (Rape, Abuse & Incest National Network). (2023). Adult survivors of child sexual abuse. Retrieved January 15, 2025, from https://www.rainn.org/articles/adult-survivors-child-sexual-abuse

The National Child Traumatic Stress Network. (2023). Sexual abuse. Retrieved January 15, 2025, from https://www.nctsn.org/what-is-child-trauma/trauma-types/sexual-abuse

Additional Reading Mentioned in Text Carnes, P. (2001). *Out of the Shadows: Understanding Sexual Addiction* (3rd ed.). Hazelden Publishing.

DeSalvo, L. (1999). *Writing as a Way of Healing: How Telling Our Stories Transforms Our Lives.* Beacon Press.

Levine, P. A. (2008). *Healing Trauma: A Pioneering Program for Restoring the Wisdom of Your Body.* Sounds True.

Maté, G. (2003). *When the Body Says No: The Cost of Hidden Stress.* Vintage Canada.

Rothschild, B. (2000). *The Body Remembers: The Psychophysiology of Trauma and Trauma Treatment.* W. W. Norton & Company.

Siegel, D. J., & Bryson, T. P. (2011). *The Whole-Brain Child: 12 Revolutionary Strategies to Nurture Your Child's Developing Mind.* Delacorte Press.

Glossary

5-4-3-2-1 GROUNDING TECHNIQUE: EMERGENCY grounding exercise where you name 5 things you can see, 4 you can touch, 3 you can hear, 2 you can smell, and 1 you can taste. Helps interrupt anxiety spirals and bring awareness to the present moment. See Chapter 1, Chapter 8, Chapter 10.

ACEs (Adverse Childhood Experiences): Potentially traumatic events that occur in childhood, such as abuse, neglect, or household dysfunction. Research shows ACEs can impact mental and physical health throughout life. Higher ACE scores correlate with increased risk for various health problems. See Chapter 19.

Adaptive Responses: Behaviors and personality traits that developed as survival strategies during trauma. They may no longer serve you in safe environments. These aren't character flaws but brilliant adaptations that can be updated as healing progresses. See Chapter 8.

Amygdala: The brain's "smoke detector" that scans for danger. After trauma, it can get stuck in "DANGER!" mode, constantly alerting to threats even in safe situations. See Introduction, Chapter 3.

Body Betrayal: When the body has physical responses during abuse, creating confusion and shame even though these biological reactions have nothing to do with consent or desire. See Chapter 3.

Body Check-ins: Regular practice of noticing physical sensations, emotions, and needs throughout the day. Helps build nervous system awareness and self-care skills. See Chapter 1, Chapter 26.

Body Memories: Physical sensations, pain, or tension that your body holds from traumatic experiences. This happens even when you don't consciously remember what happened. Your body "remembers" trauma through muscle tension, chronic pain, or specific physical reactions. See Chapter 1, Chapter 3.

Body Ownership Exercise: Somatic practice involving standing in a power pose and affirming "This is my body. I decide" to help the nervous system remember personal autonomy. See Chapter 23.

Boundaries: Limits you set to protect your physical, emotional, and mental wellbeing. Healthy boundaries help you decide what behaviors, requests, or situations you will and won't accept. They're about self-care, not punishment of others. See Chapter 16, Chapter 23.

Compartmentalization: A protective mental strategy where the mind creates separate "drawers" to store different experiences, allowing day-to-day functioning while containing traumatic material. See Chapter 3, Introduction.

Complex Trauma (C-PTSD): Trauma that results from repeated, prolonged exposure to traumatic events, especially in childhood. Unlike single-incident trauma, complex trauma affects core beliefs about self, others, and the world. It often involves emotional neglect, chronic abuse, or growing up in chaotic environments. It can shape personality development and what may seem like character traits. See Chapter 8, Chapter 19.

Coping Mechanisms: Strategies people use to manage stress, pain, or difficult emotions. They can be healthy (exercise, talking to friends) or unhealthy (self-harm, substance use). Understanding your coping patterns helps you develop healthier alternatives. See Chapter 6.

Co-regulation: The process of using another person's calm nervous system to help regulate your own. This happens naturally in healthy relationships and is essential for healing trauma. Examples include feeling calmer when sitting with a peaceful friend or having your breathing slow down when someone speaks in a soothing voice. See Chapter 17, Chapter 26.

Daily Grounding Card: A personalized list of 3-5 reliable calming tools (songs, textures, scents, movements, phrases) kept accessible for quick nervous system regulation. See Chapter 26.

Dissociation: A protective response where your mind disconnects from your body, emotions, thoughts, or surroundings during overwhelming experiences. It can range from mild "spacing out" to feeling completely outside your body. Common signs include memory gaps, feeling unreal, or watching yourself "from above." See Chapter 1, Chapter 10, Chapter 22, Chapter 23.

Emotional Dysregulation: Difficulty managing emotional responses in ways that are proportionate to the situation. It may involve intense emotions, mood swings, or feeling numb. It often results from trauma disrupting the development of healthy emotional regulation skills. See Chapter 7, Chapter 9.

Embodied Safety: The felt sense of safety in your body, not just intellectual knowledge that you're safe. This involves your nervous system actually relaxing rather than staying on high alert. It's essential for trauma healing because you can't heal while your body still believes it's in danger. See Chapter 1, Chapter 26.

Environmental Safety: Creating physical spaces and routines that signal safety to the nervous system through predictable patterns, soothing sensory input, and accessible exits. See Chapter 26.

Expanded Body Inventory: Comprehensive exercise for reconnecting with all parts of the body, including guidance for areas affected by trauma. Found in Appendix B. See Chapter 1.

Fawn Response: A survival response where you try to please others or avoid conflict to stay safe. It often develops when fighting, fleeing, or freezing aren't options. It may show up as people-pleasing, difficulty saying no, or abandoning your own needs to keep others happy. See Chapter 4, Chapter 16.

Fight Response: A survival response where your body prepares to confront danger. After trauma, this might show up as irritability, anger outbursts, or feeling aggressive when triggered. Your nervous system is trying to protect you by preparing to fight off threats. See Chapter 4.

Fight, Flight, Freeze: The three primary survival responses. Fight involves aggressive protection, flight involves escape, and freeze involves shutdown when other options aren't available. All are automatic and protective. See Introduction, Chapter 3, Chapter 4.

Flashback: Re-experiencing a traumatic event as if it's happening in the present moment. It can be emotional (feeling the same fear), physical (body reactions), visual (seeing images), or complete (feeling totally back in that moment). It's different from regular memories because flashbacks feel current and real. See Chapter 10.

Flight Response: A survival response where your body prepares to escape danger. After trauma, this might show up as anxiety, restlessness, avoiding certain places or people, or feeling like you need to constantly stay busy. See Chapter 4.

Freeze Response: A survival response where your body shuts down when fighting or fleeing isn't possible. It may involve feeling paralyzed, numb, or "playing dead." Often misunderstood as weakness, but it's actually a biological survival mechanism. See Introduction, Chapter 3, Chapter 4.

Gaslighting: A form of psychological manipulation where someone makes you question your own reality, memories, or perceptions. It often involves denying things that happened, minimizing your experiences, or making you feel "crazy" for having normal reactions. See Chapter 21.

Green Flags (in relationships): Positive signs of healthy partners who respect boundaries without question, check in about comfort and consent, handle "no" with grace, make you feel safe not anxious, and support your healing journey. See Chapter 23.

Grounding: Techniques that help bring your awareness back to the present moment and into your body when you feel triggered, anxious, or disconnected. Examples include the 5-4-3-2-1 technique, feeling your feet on the floor, or holding something with texture. See Chapter 1, Chapter 5, Chapter 8, Chapter 10.

Grooming: The process by which an abuser builds trust and breaks down defenses to prepare someone for abuse. It often involves special attention, gifts, gradually increasing boundary violations, and creating secrecy. It's designed to confuse the victim and make resistance difficult. See Chapter 2.

Hypervigilance: A state of enhanced alertness and constant scanning for potential threats. After trauma, your nervous system may stay "on guard" even in safe situations. It can be exhausting and make it difficult to relax or enjoy peaceful moments. See Chapter 3, Chapter 6, Chapter 7, Chapter 8.

Hypersexuality: Using sexual behavior to feel powerful, valuable, or in control after trauma. May involve seeking intensity because nothing else feels real or confusing sex with love. See Chapter 23.

Inner Critic: The harsh, critical voice in your head that judges, shames, or attacks you. It often develops as a way to try to prevent future harm by being "perfect" or "good enough." It can sound like an internalized version of past abusers or critical caregivers. See Chapter 24.

Inner Critic Parts: Different protective aspects that developed during trauma, including the Preemptive Striker ("I'll hurt us first so others can't"), Perfectionist Protector ("If we're perfect, we won't give them reasons"), Minimizer ("We're nothing, so expect nothing"), and Abuser's Echo (repeating the abuser's words). Each needs different healing approaches. See Chapter 24.

Internal Parts/Parts Work: The understanding that we all have different aspects or "parts" of our personality that serve protective functions. After trauma, some parts may become dominant (like people-pleasing or hypervigilant parts) and be mistaken for core personality. Healing involves recognizing and working with these parts. See Chapter 4, Chapter 5, Chapter 8.

Internal Safety: The permission and freedom to have needs, speak kindly to yourself, trust your perceptions, and exist without internal criticism or judgment. See Chapter 26.

Intrusive Thoughts: Unwanted thoughts, images, or urges that pop into your mind without your control. They're common after trauma and can include memories of abuse, self-harm thoughts, or fears about safety. Having these thoughts doesn't mean you want them or will act on them. See Chapter 10, Chapter 25.

Lauren's Story: Case study of a survivor who experienced manipulation and coercion in a teenage relationship, illustrating boundary confusion and the healing journey through therapy and self-discovery. See Chapter 23.

Mandated Reporting: Legal requirement for certain professionals (teachers, doctors, therapists, social workers, etc.) to report suspected current child abuse to authorities. Does not typically apply to adult survivors disclosing past childhood abuse when no children are currently at risk. See Chapter 27.

Nervous System: The network in your body that controls your responses to safety and danger. It includes the sympathetic system (activates fight/flight) and parasympathetic system (promotes rest and healing). After trauma, it can get stuck in "survival mode" even when you're safe. See Chapter 1, Chapter 3, Chapter 13, Chapter 26.

Nervous System Regulation: The ability to manage your body's stress responses and return to a calm state after activation. Healthy regulation allows you to respond appropriately to real threats while staying calm in safe situations. Trauma can disrupt this ability. See Chapter 1, Chapter 13.

Nervous System Safety: Teaching the body it's truly safe to let its guard down through environmental, relational, personal permission, and internal safety practices. Allows shift from "survive" to "heal" mode. See Chapter 26.

Neuroplasticity: The brain's ability to reorganize itself by forming new neural connections throughout life. This means your brain can literally rewire itself based on new experiences, thoughts, and behaviors. For trauma survivors, neuroplasticity offers hope because it shows that trauma's effects on the brain aren't permanent. Through healing practices like therapy, mindfulness, and positive relationships, you can create new neural pathways that support health and wellbeing. Your brain remains capable of change and growth regardless of your age or how long you've carried trauma. See Chapter 3, Chapter 8, Chapter 18.

Parasympathetic Nervous System: The part of your nervous system responsible for "rest and digest" functions. When activated, it promotes calm, healing, and connection. Trauma healing involves strengthening this system's ability to bring you back to baseline after stress. See Chapter 13.

Parts/Internal Parts: Different aspects of personality that develop to handle overwhelming experiences. After trauma, the mind creates separate "compartments" or parts to hold different feelings and experiences—like having different drawers for scared feelings, anger, or "everything's fine" feelings. This isn't mental illness but evidence of the mind's ability to survive impossible circumstances. See Introduction, Chapter 4, Chapter 5, Chapter 8.

Personal Permission: The freedom to say no without explanation, feel feelings without judgment, rest without guilt, and exist authentically without fear of abandonment or punishment. See Chapter 26.

Pornography (trauma complications): For survivors, pornography can create additional healing complications through early exposure trauma, unhealthy sexuality education, and compulsive use for emotional numbing. See Chapter 23.

Prefrontal Cortex: The logical, planning, "I can handle this" part of the brain that goes offline during stress, leading to foggy thinking and difficulty with decision-making after trauma. See Introduction, Chapter 3.

RAIN Technique: Four-step mindfulness practice for processing difficult emotions: Recognize what's happening, Allow the experience to be there, Investigate with kindness, and Non-attachment (not identifying with the experience). See Chapter 5, Chapter 8, Chapter 13.

Relational Safety: Relationships where you can be authentic without performing, people respect boundaries without guilt-tripping, and support is offered without requiring gratitude or being "fixed" in return. See Chapter 26.

Revictimization: The increased likelihood of experiencing additional trauma after an initial traumatic experience. It's not the victim's fault, but trauma can affect judgment, boundaries, or self-protection skills in ways that increase vulnerability. Understanding this helps with prevention and self-compassion. See Chapter 8.

Self-Compassion: Treating yourself with the same kindness you'd show a good friend who was struggling. It involves recognizing your pain, understanding that suffering is part of human experience, and responding to yourself with care rather than criticism. See Chapter 11.

Sexual Avoidance: Complete shutdown of sexual desire, physical numbness during intimacy, or panic at the thought of vulnerability as a trauma response. See Chapter 23.

Sexual Trauma Reenactment: Being drawn to partners who remind you of your abuser, recreating abusive dynamics, or seeking familiar dysfunction over unfamiliar health. See Chapter 23.

Shame: The painful feeling that you are fundamentally flawed, bad, or wrong. Different from guilt (feeling bad about what you did), shame is feeling bad about who you are. Often a core wound in sexual trauma that requires specific healing approaches. See Chapter 5, Chapter 6.

Sleep Hygiene: Practices and habits that promote good quality sleep. It includes consistent bedtimes, limiting screens before bed, creating a comfortable sleep environment, and avoiding caffeine late in the day. It's especially important for trauma survivors since sleep disturbances are common. See Chapter 10, Chapter 26.

Somatic: Relating to the body and physical sensations. Somatic approaches to trauma healing focus on body awareness and physical experiences rather than just talking about trauma. It's based on understanding that trauma is stored in the body, not just the mind. See Chapter 1, Chapter 13.

STOP Technique: Emergency intervention for freeze response: Stop what you're doing, Take a breath, Observe your body and surroundings, Proceed with intention. Helps interrupt the freeze state and restore choice. See Chapter 4.

Stuck/Trapped Energy: Survival energy (fight, flight, freeze responses) that becomes trapped in the body when escape wasn't possible during trauma. This energy transforms into symptoms like depression, anxiety, chronic pain, and other trauma responses until it can be safely released. See Introduction, Chapter 1, Chapter 4.

Survival Mode: A state where your nervous system is focused primarily on staying alive rather than learning, growing, or connecting. It involves chronic activation of stress responses (fight, flight, freeze, fawn). While helpful during actual danger, it becomes problematic when it continues after safety is restored. See Chapter 3, Chapter 10.

Sympathetic Nervous System: The part of your nervous system that activates during stress or danger, triggering fight-or-flight responses. It increases heart rate, breathing, and alertness. After trauma, this system may become overactive, leading to chronic anxiety or hypervigilance. See Chapter 13.

Three-Times Check-In: Body awareness exercise involving checking physical sensations, emotional state, and current needs. Practiced three times daily to build nervous system awareness. See Chapter 1.

Tonic Immobility: Scientific term for the freeze response during assault. An involuntary survival mechanism where the body becomes immobilized, often accompanied by dissociation. Not a choice or sign of consent. See Chapter 4.

Transition Rituals: Small practices between activities (deep breaths, stretches, affirmations) that help the nervous system move from one state to another safely. See Chapter 26.

Trauma: Not just what happened to you, but what got trapped inside you when the bad thing happened. Trauma is the stuck survival energy that had nowhere to go during overwhelming experiences. Can be a single incident or ongoing experiences that overwhelm your ability to cope. See Introduction, Chapter 3.

Trauma Adaptations: Specific behaviors, thought patterns, or personality traits that developed in response to trauma. Examples include hypervigilance, people-pleasing, emotional numbness, or perfectionism. These adaptations were protective during trauma but may limit growth in safe environments. See Chapter 8.

Trauma Amnesia: Memory loss surrounding traumatic events. It can involve forgetting parts of or entire traumatic experiences. This is a normal protective response, not a sign of weakness or lying. Memories may return gradually as healing progresses. See Chapter 22.

Trauma Bond: A strong emotional attachment that develops between an abuser and victim through cycles of abuse and positive attention. The intermittent reinforcement creates a powerful psychological bond that can be difficult to break. It's not the victim's fault or choice. See Chapter 8.

Trauma Response: Your body and mind's automatic reaction to re-minders of past trauma. It can include emotional, physical, or behav-ioral responses that feel out of proportion to the current situation. These responses made sense during the original trauma and take time to change. See Chapter 4, Chapter 10.

Trigger: Anything that reminds your brain of trauma and activates a trauma response. It can be sights, sounds, smells, sensations, situa-tions, or even internal experiences like emotions or thoughts. Triggers can be obvious or subtle, and responses can vary in intensity. See Chap-ter 10.

Two-Part Definition of Trauma: Part 1 is the violation itself (what happened), Part 2 is the ongoing impact (how the nervous system re-organized around the violation). Trauma lives primarily in the second part. See Chapter 3.

Vagus Nerve: A major nerve that connects your brain to your body and plays a key role in the parasympathetic nervous system. When func-tioning well, it helps you feel calm and connected. Trauma can disrupt its function, but specific exercises can help restore healthy vagal tone. See Chapter 13.

Watchdog Part: The hypervigilant aspect of personality that con-stantly scans for danger and evaluates threats and safety. Developed as protection during trauma but can become exhausting when constantly active. See Chapter 4, Chapter 5, Chapter 8.

Window of Tolerance: The zone where you can handle stress and strong emotions without becoming overwhelmed or shutting down. Trauma can narrow this window, making you more likely to flip into fight/flight or freeze states. Healing involves gradually expanding this window. See Chapter 7, Chapter 26.

Your Bill of Sexual Rights: List of fundamental rights including defining your own sexuality, changing your mind, saying no/yes on your terms, taking time needed, and healing at your own pace. See Chapter 23.

Your Boundary Bill of Rights: List of fundamental boundary rights that establish your authority over your own life, choices, and well-being. Includes the right to say no, change your mind, have privacy, and set limits without justification. See Chapter 16.

Your Bill of Rights: Core list of personal rights that affirm your inherent worth and autonomy. Establishes that you have the right to be treated with respect, make your own choices, and exist without having to earn your value. See Chapter 8.

Resources for Continued Healing

Crisis Support (Available 24/7)

United States

R AINN (RAPE, ABUSE & Incest National Network)

National Sexual Assault Hotline: 1-800-656-HOPE (4673)

- **Online Chat:** online.rainn.org

- **Spanish:** rainn.org/es

Crisis Text Line

- **Text HOME to:** 741741

- **WhatsApp:** +1-443-331-6102

- **Spanish:** Text AYUDA to 741741

National Suicide Prevention Lifeline

- **Call or Text:** 988

- **Chat:** 988lifeline.org/chat

National Domestic Violence Hotline

- **Phone:** 1-800-799-7233

- **Text START to:** 88788

- **Website:** thehotline.org

LGBT National Hotline

- **Phone:** 1-888-843-4564

- **Website:** lgbthotline.org

SAMHSA National Helpline (Substance Abuse)

- **Phone:** 1-800-662-4357

Canada

Crisis Services Canada

- **Phone:** 1-833-456-4566

- **Text:** 45645

- **Website:** crisisservicescanada.ca

Kids Help Phone

- **Phone:** 1-800-668-6868

- **Text:** Text CONNECT to 686868

United Kingdom

Samaritans

- **Phone:** 116 123 (free from any phone)

- **Email:** jo@samaritans.org

- **Website:** samaritans.org

Rape Crisis England & Wales

- **Phone:** 0808 802 9999

- **Website:** rapecrisis.org.uk

SupportLine

- **Phone:** 01708 765200

- **Website:** supportline.org.uk

Australia

Lifeline

- **Phone:** 13 11 14

- **Text:** 0477 13 11 14

- **Website:** lifeline.org.au

1800RESPECT (Sexual Assault)

- **Phone:** 1800 737 732

- **Website:** 1800respect.org.au

New Zealand

Lifeline

- **Phone:** 0800 543 354

- **Website:** lifeline.org.nz

Safe to Talk (Sexual Harm)

- **Phone:** 0800 044 334 **Text:** 433

- **Website:** safetotalk.nz

Ireland

Samaritans Phone:

- 116 123

- **Website:** samaritans.org

Rape Crisis Network Ireland

- **Phone:** 1800 778 888

- **Website:** rcni.ie

Spanish-Speaking Countries

Spain - Teléfono de la Esperanza

- **Phone:** 717 003 717

- **Website:** telefonodelaesperanza.org

México - SAPTEL

- **Phone:** 55 5259-8121

- **Website:** saptel.org.mx

Colombia

- **Línea de Prevención del Suicidio**

- **Phone:** 106

Argentina

- **Centro de Asistencia al Suicida**

- **Phone:** 135

Online Resources

General Support

RAINN.org Comprehensive resources, survivor stories, and local provider search

1in6.org Specifically for male survivors of sexual abuse

Male Survivor Website: malesurvivor.org - Resources and support for male survivors

Pandora's Project Website: pandys.org - Online support community

After Silence Website: aftersilence.org - Message board and chat room for survivors

The Voices and Faces Project Website: voicesandfaces.org - Survivor stories and resources

Adult Survivors of Child Abuse (ASCA) Website: ascasupport.org - Resources and meetings

7 Cups Website: 7cups.com - Free emotional support chat

International Resources

SurvivorsUK.org UK-based support for male survivors

The Blue Knot Foundation (Australia) Website: blueknot.org.au

Survivors Trust (UK) Website: thesurvivorstrust.org

Specialized Support

National Child Traumatic Stress Network Website: nctsn.org

INCITE (for BIPOC survivors) Website: incite-national.org

Partners of Survivors Website: pos-ffcsas.org - Support for partners and families

Support Organizations

National Center for Victims of Crime Website: victimsofcrime.org

Phone: 1-855-4-VICTIM (1-855-484-2846)

Childhelp National Child Abuse Hotline Phone: 1-800-4-A-CHILD (1-800-422-4453)

Darkness to Light Website: d2l.org - Prevention and response training

SNAP (Survivors Network of those Abused by Priests) Website: snapnetwork.org

The Joyful Heart Foundation Website: joyfulheartfoundation.org

GRACE (Godly Response to Abuse in Christian Environment) Website: netgrace.org

Mending the Soul Website: mendingthesoul.org - Faith-based healing resources

Sacred Survivors Website: sacred-survivors.com

Apps for Healing

Crisis Support

PTSD Coach (Free) Created by VA, helpful for all trauma survivors

notOK Crisis support app for immediate help

Mental Health

Calm Meditation, sleep stories, and mindfulness

Headspace Guided meditation and mindfulness

Insight Timer Free meditation app with large community

Sanvello Mood tracking and coping skills

Youper Emotional health assistant

Trauma-Specific

EMDR Therapy Games For trauma processing support

Breathe2Relax Breathing exercises for anxiety

Tapping Solution EFT/tapping techniques for emotional regulation

Recommended Reading

Foundational Trauma Books

- *The Body Keeps the Score* by Bessel van der Kolk, MD

- *Waking the Tiger* by Peter Levine

- *In an Unspoken Voice* by Peter Levine

- *Complex PTSD* by Pete Walker

- *Trauma and Recovery* by Judith Herman, MD

- *When the Body Says No* by Gabor Maté

- *The Myth of Normal* by Gabor Maté

For Sexual Abuse Recovery

- *The Courage to Heal* by Ellen Bass & Laura Davis

- *Victims No Longer* by Mike Lew (for male survivors)

- *The Sexual Healing Journey* by Wendy Maltz

- *Allies in Healing* by Laura Davis (for partners)

- *It's Not You, It's What Happened to You* by Christine Lang-ley-Obaugh

Body-Based Healing

- *The Body Remembers* by Babette Rothschild

- *Healing Trauma* by Peter Levine

- *The Haunted Self* by Onno Van Der Hart, Ellert R. S. Nijenhuis PhD, et al. (for dissociation)

Shame and Self-Worth

- *Healing the Shame that Binds You* by John Bradshaw

- *Rising Strong* by Brené Brown

- *Self-Compassion* by Kristin Neff

Creative Healing

- *Managing Stress with Art* by Cathy Malchiodi

- *Writing as a Way of Healing* by Louise DeSalvo

Faith-Based Resources

- *The Wounded Heart* by Dan Allender

- *Redeeming Love* by Francine Rivers (fiction)

- *When God Weeps* by Joni Eareckson Tada

Specialized Topics

- *The Boy Who Was Raised as a Dog* by Bruce Perry

- *Transcending Trauma* by Frank G. Anderson, Brian Arens, et al. (for childhood abuse)

- *My Name is Not Easy* by Debby Dahl Edwardson (Indigenous trauma)

- *Pleasure Activism* by adrienne maree brown (reclaiming body autonomy)

- *Rest is Resistance* by Tricia Hersey (trauma and rest)

Finding Professional Help

Therapist Directories

Psychology Today Website: psychologytoday.com/us/therapists

National Board for Certified Counselors Website: nbcc.org

Specialized Training Organizations

ISSTD (International Society for the Study of Trauma and Dissociation) Website: isstd.org

EMDRIA (EMDR International Association) Website: emdria.org

Somatic Experiencing International Website: traumahealing.org

American Professional Society on the Abuse of Children Website: apsac.org

What to Look For in a Therapist

When searching for professional support, look for someone with trauma-informed care training who has specific experience working with sexual abuse survivors. If you're interested in body-based approaches to healing, seek practitioners who understand somatic methods. Cultural competency matters too—find someone who understands your background and identity. Most importantly, trust your gut about whether this person feels safe and non-judgmental to you.

Important Notes

If you're in **immediate danger**, call **911** (US), **999** (UK), or your local emergency number. Online communities can be helpful but use caution about sharing personal information. Remember that healing is not linear—having bad days doesn't mean you're not making progress. You deserve support and you deserve to heal.

Remember: Recovery looks different for everyone. Use the resources that feel right for you and leave the ones that don't. You are the expert on your own healing journey.

Audio Support Available: Guided audio versions of select exercises are available at https://healingwhathidesintheshadows.com/to support your healing practice.

Complete Trauma Recovery Toolkit

All the exercises from this book organized for easy reference

Emergency Tools for Crisis Moments

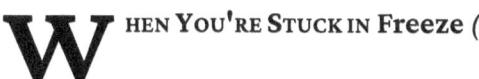

WHEN YOU'RE STUCK IN **Freeze** *(Chapter 4)*

Use when you feel:

Mind going blank

Unable to speak or find words

Disconnected from your body

Overwhelmed and shutting down

Like you want to disappear

The STOP Technique:

S - STOP whatever you're doing, just pause

T - TAKE 3 breaths slowly, make exhales longer than inhales

O - OBSERVE what's happening in your body without fixing it

P - PAUSE and give yourself permission to take time

Remember: This feeling will pass. You are safe now.

Emergency Grounding When Triggered *(Chapter 1)*

5-4-3-2-1 Grounding Technique:

5 things you can see

4 things you can touch (and touch them)

3 things you can hear

2 things you can smell

1 thing you can taste

Temperature Shock:

Hold ice cubes

Splash cold water on face

Take a hot shower

Step outside into different air

Time and Place Reminder Say out loud or write:

"My name is [your name]"

"I am [your age] years old"

"I am in [location]"

"The date is [today's date]"

"I am safe now"

Body Awareness and Reconnection

Safety Check Before Body Work *(Chapter 1)*

Ask yourself:

Am I in a private space where I won't be interrupted?

Do I have a trusted person I can contact if needed?

Can I stop this exercise at any time?

Do I have a grounding object nearby?

Permission Setting: Say: "I give myself permission to feel what I feel, or to feel nothing at all. Both are okay. I am in control of this experience."

Stage 1: External Awareness *(Chapter 1) Start here if very disconnected*

Temperature Mapping:

Notice air temperature on your skin

Compare warmth of face vs. hands

Feel air moving from breathing or fans

Pressure Points:

Press feet into floor

Squeeze hands together

Hug yourself gently

Feel chair supporting you

Movement Awareness:

Slowly move head side to side

Shrug shoulders up and down

Wiggle fingers and toes

Rock gently back and forth

Stage 2: Surface Sensations *(Chapter 1)*

Clothing Contact:

Notice where clothes touch skin

Feel texture of sleeves on arms

Notice weight of clothing

Feel shoes against feet

Skin Exploration: *For those with touch trauma: start with hands only*

Gently touch arm with opposite hand

Try light brushing, gentle pressure, circular motions

Use soft object like feather if direct touch feels unsafe

Stage 3: Internal Landscape *(Chapter 1)*

Breath as Gateway:

Place one hand on chest, one on belly

Don't change breathing, just notice

Which hand moves more?

Feel air moving in and out of nose

Heartbeat Discovery:

Place hand on chest - can you feel heartbeat?

Try fingers on wrist pulse point

Jump 10 times, then check again

If you can't feel it: This is normal with dissociation

Internal Body Scan: Go slowly through each area:

Head and face

Neck and shoulders

Arms and hands

Chest and heart

Stomach and abdomen

Pelvis and hips

Legs and feet

Notice what you feel, or notice the absence of feeling without judgment.

What You Might Experience

If You Feel Nothing:

This is not failure - numbness protects you

Say: "Thank you, body, for keeping me safe"

Try external awareness exercises

This IS progress - you're paying attention

If You Feel Too Much:

You're not broken - your system is sensitive

Use grounding: feet on floor, cold water, deep breathing

Go slower, take breaks

Remember: you can stop anytime

If Emotions Arise:

Bodies hold emotions - this is normal

Common: sadness, fear, anger

Let emotions move through you

You can feel emotions and stay safe

Breathing and Nervous System Regulation

Basic Breathing Techniques

Trauma-Informed Breath *(Chapter 13)*

Breathe naturally, just noticing

Count: in for 4, hold for 4, out for 4

If holding feels triggering: in for 4, out for 6

Place hand on chest or belly to feel movement

"Voo" Breath for Energy Release *(Chapter 4)*

Sit comfortably, take natural breath

On exhale, make low "voo" sound from belly

Let sound vibrate through body

Notice any warmth or tingling

Repeat 2-3 times, then rest

4-7-8 Breath for Calm *(Chapter 13)*

Breathe in for 4 counts

Hold for 7 counts

Breathe out for 8 counts

Movement and Energy Release

Somatic Movement Exercises

Freeze Response Shaking *(Chapter 4)*

Stand with feet hip-width apart

Begin gently bouncing knees

Let shaking travel up your body

Continue 30-60 seconds

Rest and notice sensations

Boundary Push *(Chapter 4)*

Stand with feet hip-width apart

Extend arms, palms facing out

Deep breath, exhale saying "No" while pushing forward

Feel power creating physical space

Power Pose *(Chapter 22)*

Stand with feet hip-width apart

Place hands on hips

Take deep breath and say: "This is my body. I decide."

Feel strength in your stance

Bilateral Stimulation *(Chapter 22)*

Cross arms over chest, hands on opposite shoulders

Gently tap alternating shoulders: left, right, left, right

Say internally: "I am here. I am now. I am safe."

Safety Sandwich *(Chapter 26)*

Lie down with heavy blanket under and over you

Feel pressure from above, support from below

Breathe deeply: "I am held. I am contained. I am safe."

Emotional Regulation and Release

Managing Intense Emotions

RAIN Technique for Difficult Emotions *(Chapter 7)*

Recognize: "I notice I'm feeling..."

Allow: "It's okay to feel this"

Investigate: "Where do I feel this in my body?"

Nurture: "What do I need right now?"

Ice Water Face Plunge *(Chapter 25)* When self-harm urges arise:

Fill bowl with ice water

Take deep breath and plunge face in for few seconds

Follow with gentle face drying and deep breathing

Provides intensity without damage

Movement Story:

Put on music

Let your body tell story through movement

Start curled up if needed

Let body show the journey

Writing and Expression

Therapeutic Writing Exercises

The Feeling Dump:

Set timer for 5-10 minutes

Write whatever you're feeling

Don't stop, edit, or judge

If stuck, write "I don't know what to write"

Daily Worth Evidence List *(Chapter 11)* Each day write three pieces of evidence you have worth:

Kind things you did (even tiny ones)

Challenges you faced

Positive impacts you had

"I Am / I Am Not" List:

I AM column: truths about who you really are

I AM NOT column: lies trauma wants you to believe

Truth-Flip Practice *(Chapter 24)*

Notice negative thought

Ask: "Where did I learn this?"

Challenge with evidence

Rewrite with truth

Creative Expression

Feelings Color Wheel:

Assign colors to feelings

Paint/draw with those colors when emotions arise

No need to make "things" - just let color express

Safe Space Creation:

Draw, build, or describe completely safe place

Add every detail: colors, sounds, smells

Visit mentally when overwhelmed

Identity and Self-Discovery Work

Discovering Your True Self

The Opposite Experiment (Chapter 8)

Take a "personality trait" and try its opposite in small, safe ways

Always say yes? Try saying no to something tiny

Always independent? Ask for one small favor

Always serious? Watch something silly

Notice how it feels - foreign doesn't mean wrong

Values Excavation *(Chapter 8)*

Ask: Under the trauma responses, what do I truly value?

Connection? Creativity? Peace? Justice?

Those values point to who you really are

Let values, not trauma patterns, guide choices

The Joy Detective *(Chapter 8)*

What brings you genuine joy (not just relief or numbness)?

Notice moments of authentic lightness

These are clues to your true self beneath adaptations

Parts Mapping Exercise *(Chapter 8)*

List your "personality traits" that feel limiting

For each one, ask: "What part of me acts this way?"

Consider: "How old does this part feel?"

Explore: "What was this part protecting me from?"

Thank each part: "You helped us survive"

Update gently: "Let's give you a new job description"

Somatic True Self Discovery *(Chapter 8)*

Stand with feet hip-width apart

Place one hand on heart, one on belly

Breathe deeply and ask: "Who am I beneath all the protection?"

Don't force answers - notice what arises in your body

Sometimes your true self speaks in sensations before words

Shame and Self-Worth Work

Shame Interruption Techniques

Inner Critic Silencing *(Chapter 24)*

Place one hand over mouth, one over heart

Take deep breath

As you exhale, move hand from mouth outward (removing words)

Press hand on heart (sealing in compassion)

Truth Reclaiming Exercise *(Chapter 19)*

Stand with back against wall

Press whole spine against it, feel solid support

Take three deep breaths

Step away but imagine support still with you

Shame Posture Reset *(Chapter 11)*

Notice if you're curled inward

Slowly straighten spine

Lift chest, breathe into heart space

Worth-Building Practices

Daily Worth Practice:

Place hand on heart each morning

Say: "I have worth"

Start with 10 seconds, build up

Circles of Identity *(Chapter 11)* Draw three circles inside each other:

Inner circle: your core self (creative, kind, etc.)

Middle circle: your connections and values

Outer circle: your experiences (including but not limited to trauma)

Boundary Setting and Protection

Boundary Practice Exercises

Mirror Boundary Practice *(Chapter 16)* Look yourself in the eye and practice saying:

"No"

"I don't want to"

"Stop"

"I'm not okay with that"

The 24-Hour Rule *(Chapter 16)* For any big request: "Let me think about it and get back to you tomorrow"

Broken Record Technique *(Chapter 16)* When someone pushes past your no:

"I said no"

"I said no"

"I said no"

Pre-Disclosure Grounding *(Chapter 27)*

Stand with back against wall feeling support

Take three breaths

Step away but imagine support still with you

Quick Reference: Crisis Toolkit

Triggered: 5-4-3-2-1 grounding, temperature shock, call support

Dissociating: Press feet into floor, name location/date, bilateral stimulation

Anxious: 4-7-8 breathing, collar bone tapping, movement

Shame Attack: Hand on heart, "This will pass," worth evidence list

Boundaries Crossed: Take space, broken record, "My no is complete"

Building Your Practice

Week 1-2: Foundation

Focus on external awareness and basic grounding

Practice every other day

Celebrate any sensation, however small

Week 3-4: Expansion

Add internal awareness when ready

Notice patterns: what time/position works best?

Some days you'll feel more, some less - both fine

Month 2 and Beyond:

Body awareness will fluctuate - this is normal

Use body signals for decision-making

Integrate with other healing practices

When to Seek Additional Support

Consider professional help if:

You consistently feel unsafe during exercises

Flashbacks or panic attacks occur regularly

You feel unable to sense body after several weeks

Self-harm urges arise from body awareness

You need guidance with trauma-specific areas

Important Safety Notes

Immediate danger: Call 911 (US), 999 (UK), or local emergency number

Online communities: Can be helpful but use caution sharing personal information

Healing is not linear: Bad days don't mean you're not making progress

You deserve support: And you deserve to heal

Remember: These tools are yours now. Use what helps, skip what doesn't feel right, and trust your own timing.

Audio Support Available: Guided audio versions of select exercises are available at https://healingwhathidesintheshadows.com/ to support your healing practice.

INDEX BY CHAPTER

Coaching Corners

For immediate crisis support:

National Sexual Assault Hotline: 1-800-656-HOPE (4673)

Crisis Text Line: Text HOME to 741741

National Suicide Prevention Lifeline: Call or text 988

Supplement: Who God Says You Are

*U*NCHANGEABLE *T*RUTHS *A*BOUT *Y*OUR *Identity*

No matter what was done to you, these truths about who you are in God's eyes remain unchanged and unchangeable.

You Are Loved

Loved with an everlasting love: "I have loved you with an everlasting love; I have drawn you with unfailing kindness." (Jeremiah 31:3)

Nothing can separate you from this love: "Neither height nor depth, nor anything else in all creation, will be able to separate us from the love of God." (Romans 8:39)

Loved before you did anything to earn it: "But God demonstrates his own love for us in this: While we were still sinners, Christ died for us." (Romans 5:8)

You Are Chosen and Wanted

Chosen before the world began: "For he chose us in him before the creation of the world to be holy and blameless in his sight." (Ephesians 1:4)

Wanted as His child: "See what great love the Father has lavished on us, that we should be called children of God! And that is what we are!" (1 John 3:1)

Adopted into His family: "He predestined us for adoption to sonship through Jesus Christ, in accordance with his pleasure and will." (Ephesians 1:5)

You Are Clean and Pure

Washed clean: "But you were washed, you were sanctified, you were justified in the name of the Lord Jesus Christ." (1 Corinthians 6:11)

Made new: "Therefore, if anyone is in Christ, the new creation has come: The old has gone, the new is here!" (2 Corinthians 5:17)

White as snow: "Though your sins are like scarlet, they shall be as white as snow." (Isaiah 1:18)

You Are Protected

God is your refuge: "God is our refuge and strength, an ever-present help in trouble." (Psalm 46:1)

He will never leave you: "Never will I leave you; never will I forsake you." (Hebrews 13:5)

You are held in His hands: "No one will snatch them out of my hand." (John 10:28)

You Are Valuable

Fearfully and wonderfully made: "I praise you because I am fearfully and wonderfully made; your works are wonderful." (Psalm 139:14)

Worth more than sparrows: "So don't be afraid; you are worth more than many sparrows." (Matthew 10:31)

God's treasured possession: "For you are a people holy to the Lord your God. The Lord your God has chosen you out of all the peoples on the face of the earth to be his people, his treasured possession." (Deuteronomy 7:6)

You Have Purpose

Created for good works: "For we are God's handiwork, created in Christ Jesus to do good works, which God prepared in advance for us to do." (Ephesians 2:10)

God has plans for you: "For I know the plans I have for you,' declares the Lord, 'plans to prosper you and not to harm you, plans to give you hope and a future." (Jeremiah 29:11)

Your life has meaning: "And we know that in all things God works for the good of those who love him." (Romans 8:28)

You Are Strong in Him

More than a conqueror: "In all these things we are more than conquerors through him who loved us." (Romans 8:37)

You can do all things through Christ: "I can do all this through him who gives me strength." (Philippians 4:13)

God's power works in your weakness: "My grace is sufficient for you, for my power is made perfect in weakness." (2 Corinthians 12:9)

You Are Free

Set free from shame: "There is therefore now no condemnation for those who are in Christ Jesus." (Romans 8:1)

Free indeed: "So if the Son sets you free, you will be free indeed." (John 8:36)

No longer a slave to fear: "The Spirit you received does not make you slaves, so that you live in fear again; rather, the Spirit you received brought about your adoption to sonship." (Romans 8:15)

You Are Never Alone

God is with you: "Be strong and courageous. Do not be afraid or terrified because of them, for the Lord your God goes with you; he will never leave you nor forsake you." (Deuteronomy 31:6)

He is close to the brokenhearted: "The Lord is close to the brokenhearted and saves those who are crushed in spirit." (Psalm 34:18)

Nothing can snatch you away: "I give them eternal life, and they shall never perish; no one will snatch them out of my hand." (John 10:28)

You Are Being Renewed

He is making all things new: "He who was seated on the throne said, 'I am making everything new!'" (Revelation 21:5)

Being transformed: "And we all, who with unveiled faces contemplate the Lord's glory, are being transformed into his image with ever-increasing glory." (2 Corinthians 3:18)

He completes what He starts: "Being confident of this, that he who began a good work in you will carry it on to completion until the day of Christ Jesus." (Philippians 1:6)

Reclaiming Sacred Story: A Writing Exercise

Using Scripture as a framework for processing pain and finding hope.

Choose a Biblical narrative that resonates with your experience:

For feeling abandoned: Psalm 22 ("My God, my God, why have you forsaken me?")

For betrayal: David and Bathsheba, or Jesus and Judas

For family trauma: Joseph and his brothers

For feeling unclean: The woman with the issue of blood (Mark 5:25-34)

For powerlessness: Tamar's story (2 Samuel 13) - handled with great care

For restoration: The Prodigal Son, or Hosea and Gomer

The Writing Process:

Step 1: Read the passage slowly, noting what resonates with your experience.

Step 2: Write yourself into the story. Put yourself in the scene. What do you see, hear, feel? Where are you in relation to the main character?

Step 3: Have a conversation with God as present in that story. In Joseph's prison, in David's palace, beside the bleeding woman in the crowd.

Step 4: Write God's response to your presence in that story. What does God see when He looks at you there? What does He want you to know?

Sample with Psalm 22:

"God, I'm here with David, feeling abandoned like he did. The words 'why have you forsaken me' feel like my words too. I felt forsaken when [my trauma happened]. David felt you were far from saving him—I've felt that too...

[Continue writing, letting God speak into David's story and yours]"

A Personal Prayer

If you'd like, you can make these truths personal through prayer:

"God, help me believe what You say about me more than what my trauma says. When shame whispers that I'm ruined, remind me that I'm renewed. When fear says I'm alone, help me feel Your presence. When memories say I'm worthless, let Your truth drown out the lies. I may not feel these truths yet, but I choose to trust that Your word is more reliable than my feelings. Help me see myself through Your eyes—loved, chosen, clean, and precious. Amen."

Remember: These truths were written about you before you were born. They were true before anyone hurt you. They remained true while you were being hurt. They are true now. And they will be true forever. Nothing that happened to you has the power to change who God says you are.

Remember: These tools are yours to use however helps most. You don't have to perfect them. Just practicing them is healing in action.